Advances in Understanding Aortic Diseases

Teruhisa Kazui · Shinichi Takamoto
Editors

Advances in Understanding Aortic Diseases

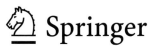

Editors:
Teruhisa Kazui, M.D.
Cardio-vascular Center
 Hokkaido Ohno Hospital
4-1Nishino, Nishi-ku
Sapporo 063-0034
Japan

Shinichi Takamoto, M.D.
Department of Cardiothoracic Surgery
Graduate School of Medicine
The University of Tokyo
7-3-1 Hongo, Bunkyo-ku
Tokyo 113-8655
Japan

ISBN: 978-4-431-99236-3   e-ISBN: 978-4-431-99237-0
DOI: 10.1007/978-4-431-99237-0
Springer Tokyo Berlin Heidelberg New York

Library of Congress Control Number: 2009925501

© Springer 2009
This work is subject to copyright. All rights are reserved, whether the whole or part of the material is concerned, specifically the rights of translation, reprinting, reuse of illustrations, recitation, broadcasting, reproduction on microfilms or in other ways, and storage in data banks.
The use of registered names, trademarks, etc. in this publication does not imply, even in the absence of a specific statement, that such names are exempt from the relevant protective laws and regulations and therefore free for general use.
Product liability: The publisher can give no guarantee for information about drug dosage and application thereof contained in this book. In every individual case the respective user must check its accuracy by consulting other pharmaceutical literature.

Printed on acid-free paper

Springer is part of Springer Science+Business Media (www.springer.com)

Preface

Thoracic aortic surgery has recently made major advances, and, as a consequence, there have been significant improvements in its outcomes. Moreover, new technologies such as endovascular treatment and diagnostic imaging with 3D-CT, MRI, and US, as well as research on the fundamental mechanism of the genesis of aortic aneurysms, are making encouraging progress.

The first international symposium on Advances in Understanding Aortic Diseases (AUAD) was convened in Europe, and subsequent symposia were shared between Europe and the United States. The first to be held in Asia was the 8th symposium, for which the venue was Tokyo, and which took place October 13–14, 2007. Because aortic diseases, especially thoracic aortic diseases, are more common in Japan than in Western countries, the arrival of the AUAD international symposium in Japan was an occasion of some significance.

In the 8th AUAD symposium, our intention was to promote further international understanding of aortic diseases, especially in Asia. The approximately 200 participants included 22 international guests, and 66 papers were presented. These proceedings contain all the papers presented in Tokyo in both the oral and the poster sessions.

I expect these proceedings to promote a greatly improved understanding, both of aortic diseases and of the current status of research into these diseases, not only here but far beyond these shores as well.

The symposium was held in conjunction with the 15th annual meeting of the Japanese Society for Aortic Surgery, for whose cooperation I would like to extend sincere thanks. In addition, I wish to express my deep appreciation to the many Japanese companies that supported the symposium, and to all the Japanese academic societies, such as the Japanese Association for Thoracic Surgery, the Japanese Society for Cardiovascular Surgery, the Japan Surgery Society, and the Japanese Circulation Society, that gave us invaluable support.

8th International Symposium on AUAD
Co-chairmen
Teruhisa Kazui
Shinichi Takamoto

The 8th Annual International Symposium on Advances
in Understanding Aortic Diseases
Joint Symposium with The 15th Annual Meeting of The Japanese
Society for Aortic Surgery
October 13 – 14, 2007
Keio Plaza Hotel, Tokyo, Japan

Organizing Committees
- Chairpersons:
  Teruhisa Kazui, M.D.
  Shinichi Takamoto, M.D.
- Committee Members:
  Hiroshi Shigematsu, M.D.
  Koichi Tabayashi, M.D.
  Sachio Kuribayashi, M.D.
  Takao Ohki, M.D.

Faculty Members

Hideo Adachi
Motomi Andou
Shigeyuki Aomi
Shigeaki Aoyagi
Tetsuya Higami
Kiyotaka Imoto
Shin Ishimaru
Tsuyoshi Itoh
Souichiro Kitamura
Tetsuo Kumazaki
Shunei Kyo
Masunori Matsuzaki

Tetsuro Miyata
Hitoshi Ogino
Kuni Ohtomo
Taijiro Sueda
Toru Suzuki
Kuniyoshi Tanaka
Ryuji Tominaga
Yuichi Ueda
Keishu Yasuda
Kiyoshi Yoshida
Ryohei Yozu

Secretariat
Department of Cardiothoracic Surgery
Graduate School of Medicine, The University of Tokyo
7-3-1 Hongo, Bunkyo-ku, Tokyo 113-8655, Japan
Phone: +81-3-5800-9155
Secretary: Tetsuro Morota, Kan Nawata

Acknowledgements

Alfresa Pharma Corporation
ALOKA CO., LTD.
Amgen Limited
Asahi Kasei Pharma
ASKA Pharmaceutical. Co., Ltd.
Astellas Pharma Inc.
AstraZeneca K.K.
BANYU PHARMACEUTICAL CO., LTD.
Bayer Yakuhin, Ltd.
Boston Scientific Japan K.K.
Bristol-Mayers K.K.
Century Medical, Inc.
Chugai Pharmaceutical Co., Ltd.
COOK Japan Inc.
COSMOTEC Corporation
CSL Behring K.K.
DAIICHI SANKYO COMPANY, LIMITED
Dainippon Sumitomo Pharma Co., Ltd.
Edwards Lifesciences Limited
Eiken Chemical Co., Ltd.
Eisai Co., Ltd.
Eli Lilly Japan K.K.
Elmed Eisai Co., Ltd.
FUKUDA DENSHI, Co., Ltd.
Fuso Pharmaceutical Industries, Ltd.
GE Yokogawa Medical Systems, Ltd.
GlaxoSmithKline K.K.
Hama Medical Industrial Co., Ltd.
HEIWA BUSSAN CO., LTD.
JAPAN GORE-TEX INC.
Japan Lifeline Co., Ltd.
Japan Tobacco Inc.
JMS Co., Ltd.

Johnson & Johnson K.K.
Kaken Pharmaceutical Co., Ltd.
KAKEN SHOYAKU CO., LTD.
Kirin Pharma Company, Limited
Kissei Pharmaceutical Co., Ltd.
Kowa Shinyaku Company, Ltd.
Kracie Pharma, Ltd.
KYORIN PHARMACEUTICAL CO., LTD.
KYOWA HAKKO KOGYO Co., Ltd.
Maruho Co., Ltd.
Maruishi Pharmaceutical. Co., Ltd.
MEDICAL PROGRESS LIMITED
MEDICEO MEDICAL CO., LTD.
MEDICO'S HIRATA Inc.
Medtronic Japan Co., Ltd.
MEIJI SEIKA KAISHA, LTD.
Merck
Minophagen Pharmaceutical. Co., LTD.
Mitsubishi Pharma Corporation
Mitsubishi Tanabe Pharma Corporation
MOCHIDA PHARMACEUTICAL CO., LTD.
NIHON PHARMACEUTICAL CO., LTD.
Nippon Boehringer Ingelheim Co., Ltd.
Nippon Chemiphar Co., Ltd.
NIPPON KAYAKU CO., LTD.
NIPPON SHINYAKU CO., LTD.
Nippon Zoki Pharmaceutical Co., Ltd.
NIPRO CORPORATION
NIPRO PHARMA CORPORATION
Novartis Pharma K.K.
ONO PHARMACEUTICAL CO., LTD.
Otsuka Pharmaceutical Co., Ltd.
Otsuka Pharmaceutical Factory, Inc.
Paramedic Co., Ltd.
Pfizer Japan Inc.
Philips Electronics Japan, Ltd.
ROHTO Pharmaceutical Co., Ltd.
sanofi-aventis K.K.
Santen Pharmaceutical Co., Ltd.
SANWA KAGAKU KENKYUSHO CO., LTD.
SATO PHARMACEUTICAL CO., LTD.
Sawai Pharmaceutical Co., Ltd.
Schering-Plough K.K.
SENKO MEDICAL INSTRUMENT MANUFACTURING CO., LTD.
Shionogi & Co., Ltd.

SSP CO., LTD.
St. Jude Medical Japan Co., Ltd.
TAIHO Pharmaceutical Co., Ltd.
Taisho Pharmaceutical Co., Ltd.
Takeda Pharmaceutical Company Limited
Tanabe Seiyaku Co., Ltd.
TEIJIN PHARMA LIMITED
TERUMO CORPORATION
TOA EIYO LTD.
Torii Pharmaceutical Co., Ltd.
TOSHIBA MEDICAL SYSTEMS CORPORATION
TOWA PHARMACEUTICAL CO., LTD.
TOYAMA CHEMICAL CO., LTD.
TSUMURA & Co.
Tyco Helthcare Japan Inc.
VITAL Corporation
WAKAMOTO PHARMACEUTICAL CO., LTD.
Wyeth Japan
YAKULT HONSHA CO., LTD.

Contents

Lecture 1   Recent Advances in Imaging Aortic Diseases

Advances in Imaging Aortic Disease 3
Geoffrey D. Rubin

Advanced Understanding and Consensus on IMH / PAU 5
David M. Williams

Recent Advances in Imaging Aortic Diseases 7
Marek P. Ehrlich and Christian Loewe

Noninvasive Diagnosis of the Artery of Adamkiewicz 15
Kunihiro Yoshioka, Ryoichi Tanaka, and Shigeru Ehara

Lecture 2   Novel Technologies in Diagnosis and Treatment for Aortic Diseases

Gene Analysis of Marfan Syndrome 23
Naomichi Matsumoto

Evolving Medical Therapy for Abdominal Aortic Aneurysms 29
Rajdeep Deb, Hosaam H. Nasr, Ranjeet Brar,
and Matthew M. Thompson

**Regression of Abdominal Aortic Aneurysms
through Pharmacologic Therapy** 43
Koichi Yoshimura, Hiroki Aoki, Yasuhiro Ikeda, Akira Furutani,
Kimikazu Hamano, and Masunori Matsuzaki

**Gene Therapy for Treating Abdominal Aortic Aneurysm using
Chimeric Decoy Oligodeoxynucleotides Against NFκB
and ets in a Rabbit Model** 51
Takashi Miyake

Simulation Study of Aortic Valve Function Using the Fluid-structure Interaction Finite Element Method 53
Seiryo Sugiura, Susumu Katayama, Nobuyuki Umetani, and Toshiaki Hisada

Symposium 1   State of Arts: Stent Graft for Thoracic Aorta

Long Term Results of Aortic Arch Repair Using Stent Grafting Technique 63
Masaaki Kato, Kazuo Shimamura, Toru Kuratani, Hiroshi Takano, and Nobukazu Ohkubo

Endovascular Repair of Thoracic Aortic Aneurysms 65
Katsuhiko Oka

Current Endograft Therapy of Type B Aortic Dissection 67
Sidney L. Kahn and Michael D. Dake

Endovascular Treatment of Chronic Type B Aortic Dissection 79
Rossella Fattori

Long-term Evolution of Type B Dissection and Endovascular Therapy Indications 81
Arturo Evangelista, Rio Aguilar, Teresa González-Alujas, Patricia Mahia, and José Rodríguez-Palomares

Symposium 2   Brain Protection in Aortic Arch Surgery

Spinal Cord Perfusion and Protection During Surgical and Endovascular Treatment of Descending Thoracic and Thoracoabdominal Aortic Aneurysms 95
Eva B. Griepp and Randall B. Griepp

Brain Protection in Aortic Arch Surgery 103
Eva B. Griepp and Randall B. Griepp

Tools and Tricks in Monitoring the Brain During Arch Surgery 111
Marc Schepens

Brain Protection in Aortic Surgery–Antegrade Selective Cerebral Perfusion 113
Teruhisa Kazui

Intermittent Pressure Augmented Retrograde Cerebral Perfusion 121
Shinichi Takamoto, Kan Nawata, Tetsuro Morota, Kazuo Kitahori, and Mitsuhiro Kawata

Contents

**Modified Arch First Technique for Total Arch Replacement
using Hypothermic Circulatory Arrest and Retrograde
Cerebral Perfusion** 123
Yuichi Ueda

**Symposium 3 State of Arts: Treatment for Thoracoabdominal
and Abdominal Aorta**

Endovascular Repair for Thoracoabdominal Aortic Aneurysms 133
Toru Kuratani, Yukitoshi Shirakawa, Kazuo Shimamura,
Mugiho Takeuchi, Goro Matsumiya, and Yoshiki Sawa

**Multicenter Clinical trial of Zenith AAA Endovascular Graft
for Abdominal Aortic Aneurysm in Japan** 135
Kimihiko Kichikawa, Shoji Sakaguchi, Wataru Higashiura,
and Hideo Uchida

**Panel Discussion 1 Advanced Understanding
and Consensus on IMH/PAU**

Advanced Understanding and Consensus on IMH/PAU 139
Sachio Kuribayashi

Recent Advances in Imaging Aortic Diseases 141
David M. Williams

**Intramural Hematoma and Penetrating Ulcer:
VIII International Symposium on Advances
in Understanding Aortic Diseases Tokyo, 2007** 143
Thoralf M. Sundt, III

Therapeutic Strategy of Acute Aortic Intramural Hematoma 155
Shuichiro Kaji

Panel Discussion 2 What's New in Aortic Root Reimplantation?

**What's New in Aortic Root Reimplantation?: The Valsalva
Graft Design in its Anatomical Reconstruction of the Aortic Root** 165
Ruggero De Paulis, Raffaele Scaffa, Daniele Maselli,
Alessandro Bellisario, and Andrea Salica

**Expanding Indications for Valve Sparing
Procedures in Aortic Root Replacement** 173
Yutaka Okita, Masamichi Matsumori, Kenji Okada, Yoshihisa Morimoto,
Mitsuru Asano, Hiroshi Munakata, Naoto Morimoto, Hiroaki Takahashi,
and Akiko Tanaka

Poster Session 1   Aortic Dissection, Marfan Syndrome

Sivelestat Sodium is Effective to Prevent Acute Lung Injury in Acute Aortic Dissection 187
Yasushige Shingu, Norihiko Shiiya, Suguru Kubota, Yuji Naito, Kinya Matsui, Satoru Wakasa, Hiroshi Sugiki, Tsuyoshi Tachibana, Tomoji Yamakawa, Toshifumi Murashita, and Yoshiro Matsui

Long-Term Results of Emergency Prosthetic Vascular Graft Replacement for Acute Stanford A Aortic Dissection 189
Sunao Watanabe, Kohei Abe, Manabu Yamazaki, Kazufumi Ohmori, and Hitoshi Koyanagi

Perioperative Risk Factors for Hospital Mortality in Patients with Acute Type A Aortic Dissection 195
Masashi Tanaka, Naoyuki Kimura, Hideo Adachi, Atsushi Yamaguchi, and Takashi Ino

Influence of Patent False Lumen on Secondary Dilation of the Distal Aorta Following Surgery for Acute Type A Aortic Dissection 197
Naoyuki Kimura, Masashi Tanaka, Hideo Adachi, Atsushi Yamaguchi, and Takashi Ino

Penetrating Atherosclerotic Ulcer Causing Cardiac Tamponade – A Case Suggesting the Etiology of Intramural Hematoma 199
Nobuhiko Mukohara, Masato Yoshida, Satoshi Tobe, and Takashi Azami

Outcome of Patients with Acute Aortic Intramural Hematoma in the Extremely Early Stage 201
Hideyasu Kohshoh, Hideaki Yoshino, Hisashi Shimizu, Yasuhiro Ieizumi, Tatsuo Kikuchi, Takumi Inami, Wataru Nagai, Kenji Shida, Kenichi Sudo, and Yoshihiro Yamaguchi

Borderline Mesenteric Ischemia Caused by Acute Aortic Dissection: Borderline Mesenteric Ischemia in Aortic Dissection 203
Kazumasa Orihashi, Taijiro Sueda, Kenji Okada, and Katsuhiko Imai

Validity of Using Ghent Criteria for Japanese Population Suspected of Marfan Syndrome 207
Koichi Akutsu, Hiroko Morisaki, Takayuki Morisaki, Hitoshi Ogino, Masashiro Higashi, Shingo Sakamoto, Tsuyoshi Yoshimuta, Kazuya Okajima, Hiroshi Nonogi, and Satoshi Takeshita

Contents

Three Cases of Total Aortic Replacement for Marfan Syndrome 209
Eiichiro Inagaki, Sohei Hamanaka, Hisao Masaki, Masao Nakata,
Atsushi Tabuchi, Yasuhiro Yunoki, Katsuhiko Shimizu, Yuji Hirami,
Hitoshi Minami, Hiroshi Kubo, Takuro Yukawa, and Kazuo Tanemoto

**Aortic Operations in 150 Patients with Marfan Syndrome:
Tokyo Experience** 211
Takashi Azuma, Shigeyuki Aomi, Masayuki Miyagishima,
Hideyuki Tomioka, Satoshi Saito, Kenji Yamazaki, Akihiko Kawai,
and Hiromi Kurosawa

**Poster Session 2   Extensive Surgery, Root, Arch and
                    Therocoabdomonal Aorta**

Surgery for Extensive Thoracic Aortic Aneurysm 215
Hiroshi Munakata, Kenji Okada, Akiko Tanaka, Masamichi Matsumori,
Mitsuru Asano, Yoshihisa Morimoto, and Yutaka Okita

Surgical Strategy in Aortic Lesion for Marfan Syndrome 221
Akiko Tanaka, Kenji Okada, Hiroshi Munakata,
Masamichi Matsumori, and Yutaka Okita

**One-stage Repair of Total Descending Aorta
for Extended Pathologies** 225
Tetsuro Morota, Shinichi Takamoto, Tetsufumi Yamamoto,
Kan Nawata, and Mitsuhiro Kawata

**Surgical Results of Descending Thoracic and Thoracoabdominal
Aortic Aneurysm Repair Using deep Hypothermic
Circulatory Arrest** 231
Kazuhiro Naito, Masashi Tanaka, Hideo Adachi,
Atsushi Yamaguchi, and Takashi Ino

**Simultaneous Surgery for Thoracic Aortic Aneurysm with
Coronary Artery Disease** 233
Akihito Matsushita, Tatsuhiko Komiya, Nobushige Tamura,
Genichi Sakaguchi, Taira Kobayashi, Tomokuni Furukawa,
Gengo Sunagawa, and Takashi Murashita

**Svensson's (Modified Bentall) Technique using a
Long Interposed Graft for Left Coronary Artery Reconstruction** 239
Atsushi Nakahira, Yasuyuki Sasaki, Hidekazu Hirai,
Masanori Sakaguchi, Manabu Motoki, Shinsuke Kotani,
Koji Hattori, Toshihiko Shibata, and Shigefumi Suehiro

Protective Effect on Preserved Aortic Valve Cusps of Reconstructed Pseudosinuses in the Aortic Root Reimplantation Technique 241
Kan Nawata, Shinichi Takamoto, Kansei Uno, Aya Ebihara, Tetsuro Morota, Minoru Ono, and Noboru Motomura

Modified Arch First Technique Using a Trifercated Graft 247
Seiichiro Wariishi, Hideaki Nishimori, Takashi Fukutomi, Kentaro Hirohashi, and Shiro Sasaguri

Atypical Arch Replacement: Reconstruction of Four Arch Vessels and Usefulness of Arch First Method with Combined Cerebral Perfusion 249
Takayuki Uchida, Hiromi Ando, Toru Yasutsune, Toshiro Iwai, Fumio Fukumura, and Jiro Tanaka

Distal Aortic Perfusion and Cerebrospinal Fluid Drainage for Thoracoabdominal Aortic Repair 255
Shinichi Suzuki, Kiyotaka Imoto, Keiji Uchida, Kensuke Kobayashi, Kouichiro Date, Motohiko Gouda, Toshiki Hatsune, Makoto Okiyama, Takayuki Kosuge, Yutaka Toyoda, and Munetaka Masuda

Selective Reconstruction of Preoperatively Identified Adamkiewicz Artery During Descending and Thoracoabdominal Aortic Aneurysm Repair; What we have Learned 263
Satoshi Saito, Shigeyuki Aomi, Hideyuki Tomioka, Masayuki Miyagishima, and Hiromi Kurosawa

Poster Session 3   Miscellaneous

Three-stage Monitoring for Prevention of Cerebral Malperfusion During Cardiovascular Surgery 267
Kazumasa Orihashi, Taijiro Sueda, Kenji Okada, and Katsuhiko Imai

Induction of Phosphorylated BAD in Motor Neurons After Transient Spinal Cord Ischemia in Rabbits 271
Masahiro Sakurai, Koji Abe, Yasuto Itoyama, and Koichi Tabayashi

Modifying Anastomotic Site in Thoracic Aortic Surgery by Using Biodegradable Felt Strips With or Without Basic Fibroblast Growth Factor 277
Hidenori Fujiwara, Yoshikatsu Saiki, Katsuhiko Oda, Satoshi Kawatsu, Ichiro Yoshioka, Naoya Sakamoto, Toshiro Ohashi, Masaaki Sato, Yasuhiko Tabata, and Koichi Tabayashi

Late Outcome of Extra-anatomic Bypass for Infected Abdominal Aortic Aneurysm 279
Atsushi Tabuchi, Hisao Masaki, Yasuhiro Yunoki, Takuro Yukawa, Hiroshi Kubo, Eiichiro Inagaki, Sohei Hamanaka, and Kazuo Tanemoto

The Efficacy of a Bionic Baroreflex System in an Abdominal Aortic Aneurysm Surgery 281
Hideaki Nishimori, Takashi Fukutomi, Seiichiro Wariishi, Masaki Yamamoto, and Shiro Sasaguri

A Case of Two Inflammatory Aortic Aneurysms Showing Spontaneous Improvement of the First Aneurysm During Development of the Second One 283
Yuiichi Tamori, Koichi Akutsu, Tsuyoshi Yoshimuta, Shingo Sakamoto, Toshiya Okajima, Masahiro Higashi, Hitoshi Ogino, Hiroshi Nonogi, and Satoshi Takeshita

Tubercular Pseudoaneurysms of Aorta and its Branches 285
Shiv Kumar Choudhary, Sachin Talwar, Balram Airan, Srikrishna Reddy, and Sanjeev Sharma

Strategy for Treating Aneurysms in the Distal: Arch Aorta-open Surgery and Endovascular Repair with Single-branched Inoue Stent-graft 287
Hideyuki Shimizu, Naritaka Kimura, Misato Kobayashi, Nobuko Tano, Yasuko Miyaki, Tatsuo Takahashi, Kentaro Yamabe, Subaru Hashimoto, Yukio Kuribayashi, Kanji Inoue, and Ryohei Yozu

Redo Left Thoracotomy for Surgical Repair on the Descending Thoracic and Thoracoabdominal Aorta 291
Kenji Minatoya, Hitoshi Ogino, Hitoshi Matsuda, Hiroaki Sasaki, Hiroshi Tanaka, and Soichiro Kitamura

Lecture 1
Recent Advances in Imaging Aortic Diseases

Advances in Imaging Aortic Disease

Geoffrey D. Rubin

Effective therapeutic intervention, be it through open repair or endovascular means, necessitates accurate characterization of the anatomic extent of aortic abnormalities, involvement of the aortic root and aortic branches, and associated impact on end organ perfusion. Imaging using transesophageal echocardiography, magnetic resonance, and computed tomography (CT) have been key tools in aortic disease characterization. While all three modalities continue to advance and evolve, CT has undergone the most rapid evolution in recent years with the introduction of faster gantry rotation times and greater numbers of detector rows that together improve the temporal resolution of the technique and make high spatial resolution cardiac gated acquisitions of the aorta possible. This advance has been most important in the assessment of the aortic root. Gated CT angiography provides and effective means of assessing the coronary arteries, the aortic annulus and the valve leaflets. The volumetric acquisition with isotropic spatial resolution allows characterization of the complex and non-planar anatomic relationships that are prevalent when the aortic root is involved with aortic aneurysm or dissection.

While clinical imaging has focused primarily on anatomic and morphologic characterization of aortic diseases, including their impact on aortic flow, techniques are emerging that promise to provide important insights into aortic wall physiology and biology. Techniques permitting in vivo sensing of inflammation, apoptosis, cell trafficking, and gene expression are currently under investigation in animal models. Although the field of molecular imaging is in its earliest stages and practical in vivo human imaging techniques may be years away, the development of these techniques in appropriate animal models should substantially advance our understanding of aortic disease pathogenesis and progression. This presentation will aim to balance current and near-term clinical advances in CT with an introduction to the nascent field of molecular aortic imaging.

G.D. Rubin (✉)
Stanford University

Advanced Understanding and Consensus on IMH / PAU

David M. Williams

The literature on IMH and PAU presents a glaring anomaly. Both diagnoses in current practice rely almost solely on imaging criteria, yet publications of large case series rarely show imaging findings on more than 3 or 4 subjects. Furthermore, the selected images, which the journal editor must presume to be carefully chosen as representative, can often be challenged as inconclusive. What one author will call a "giant penetrating ulcer" another will call an ulcer-like projection arising from IMH. The growing dominance of endovascular over open repair ensures that pathological specimens will become even rarer. This inability to anchor etiological terms like "atherosclerotic" on confirmatory pathological specimens encourages a pragmatic approach to the acute aortic syndromes. This talk will argue that the acute aortic syndromes entail the interplay of 3 distinct factors:

(1) Initiating event: intramural hemorrhage, whether superficial due to plaque rupture or deep due to vasa vasorum rupture;
(2) Environmental modulators: propagation (of intramural hemorrhage), facilitated by intrinsic medial disease such as Marfan syndrome or resisted by severe atherosclerosis; and
(3) Random complication: development of intimal defects.

Similarly, treatment strategies can be tailored according to 3 anatomical categories of patient presentation:

(1) intramural hemorrhage without intimal defect,
(2) intramural hemorrhage with intimal defect, and
(3) intimal defect without intramural hemorrhage.

D.M. Williams (✉)
Professor of Radiology, University of Michigan Medical School, Ann Arbor, MI

Recent Advances in Imaging Aortic Diseases

Marek P. Ehrlich and Christian Loewe

Summary Acute thoracic aortic syndromes represent a spectrum of different pathologies with acute chest pain with a high risk of aortic rupture and sudden death. These include nontraumatic disease entities of the thoracic aorta, namely, dissection, intramural haematoma, penetrating atherosclerotic ulcer and aneurysm rupture. All these syndromes need fast and reliable diagnostic assessment. Transoesophageal echocardiography (TOE) and computed tomography (CT), affords important diagnostic possibilities and very interesting future perspectives. Most of these clinical findings need surgical intervention with replacement of the diseased aorta. On the other hand, especially in the last decade, endovascular techniques have evolved as a new non-invasive therapeutic option for the management of descending aortic disease.

Keywords Aorta · CT · TEE · Stentgraft

Introduction

Acute thoracic aortic syndromes encompass a spectrum of emergencies presenting with acute chest pain and marked by a high risk of aortic rupture and sudden death. These include nontraumatic disease entities of the thoracic aorta, namely, dissection, intramural haematoma, penetrating atherosclerotic ulcer and aneurysm rupture. Conventional surgical intervention on the ascending aorta and/or arch is still the method of choice and even with the introduction of profound hypothermic circulatory arrest and additional cerebral protective techniques, still a formidable

M.P. Ehrlich and C. Loewe (✉)
Department of Cardiothoracic Surgery and *Interventional Radiology
Med. Univ. of Vienna Austria, Europe

undertaken in cardiac surgery. On the other hand, endovascular techniques have revolutionized the management of descending thoracic aortic disease, with the benefit of exclusion of the pathologically altered aorta without direct surgical exposure.

In clinical practice, the most frequent imaging procedure used in the diagnostic assessment of these diseases is transoesophageal echocardiography (TOE), computed tomography (CT), which, thanks to recent technological developments [multidetector-row computed tomography (MDCT)], affords important diagnostic possibilities and very interesting future perspectives [1–4].

There are some few important questions that a cardiac surgeon needs to know:

1) Does the patient have a dissection?
2) Is the ascending aorta involved?
3) Extension of the dissection, involvement of branch vessels? Malperfusion of organs?
4) Aortic valve – stenosis – insufficiency

Historical Background

Nine years after its introduction, spiral or helical CTA is being embraced as an important noninvasive tool for imaging the thoracic aorta and its branches. The high degree of accessibility and ease with which the studies are performed make it a viable alternative to aortography. Once familiar with the principles of CTA, the acquisition phase of the examination can be completed in as little as 15 minutes.

Major Advantages

- CT angiography is fast
- CT angiography is available
- CT angiography can easily be performed in severely ill patients
- CT angiography provides sufficient spatial resolution

Examination Technique

CT angiography of the aorta requires thin sections and optimisation of the contrast-medium (CM) injection to ensure maximal enhancement of the vascular territory to be examined. Use of the smallest detector to obtain thin sections results in reduced signal-to-noise (SNR) ratio and lower image resolution, which can be corrected by increasing the exposure dose. CM administration needs to be tailored to the individual patient to ensure a constantly high level of vessel opacification. The main points in CT angiography of the aorta are:

- Unenhanced scans should always be included, as they provide a good depiction of important findings, such as endoluminal calcification and intramural haematoma hyperattenuation
- The length of the volume to be examined is assessed on the scanogram, which may be integrated by low-dose unenhanced scans
- The start of volumetric scans is synchronised with peak enhancement through the use of specific programmes (bolus test/bolus triggering)
- The scan parameters are dependent on volume length and volumetric scan duration
- The CM administration protocol is pre-established and based on the patient's weight and possible abnormalities in kidney function
- The images are subsequently reviewed interactively and reconstructed with different programmes [maximum intensity projection (MIP), shaded surface display (SSD), volume rendering (VR)]

Acquisition Technique

Unenhanced phase in a patient with suspected acute aortic disease, the unenhanced examination is crucial because it depicts key findings, such as endoluminal calcification or fresh blood in the aortic wall, the only sign of intramural haematoma. Because extensive areas may be involved, the scans can be acquired with greater thickness (4 × 5 mm). In addition, unenhanced scans may help establish whether an aortic aneurysm involves the thoracic and/or abdominal aorta and whether CT angiography can be limited to one district only. With regard to the volume length to be examined, it does not constitute a limit for MDCT. However, it should be kept to the minimum to reduce examination times and collimation, improve spatial resolution and optimise total CM dose and exposure dose.

Duration of Examination

CT angiography is performed during an inspiratory breathhold, which should never exceed 30 s. critically ill patients should be connected to an oxygen mask. Images obtained during the bolus test will usually provide a good indication of patient compliance.

If a 4-slice MDCT scanner is used, a detector configuration of 4 × 1.25 mm should be preselected; Sixteen-slice MDCT allows a thicker collimation (16 × 0.5–1.25 mm), which substantially reduces scan time by a factor of four (10–15 s).

Contrast-medium Flow Rate and Volume

The CM administration protocol (nonionic CM at a concentration of 370 mgI/ml and flow rate of 3–4 ml/s) is defined on the basis of the patient's weight (2 ml/kg of body weight) up to a maximum total volume of 150 ml. Total volume is reduced in the presence of abnormal kidney function. The goal of CM injection is to obtain a constant and sufficiently long phase of aortic opacification during which data can be acquired. Arterial enhancement is related to the flow of opacified blood travelling through the pulmonary circulation and then flowing into the aorta.

Circulation Time

In CT angiography, if the patient's circulation time is constant, the CM injection interval can be matched with the acquisition interval. Precise evaluation can be obtained by setting the start time during the first passage of the entire bolus using bolus tracking. The method is based on a series of sequential automatic measurements of attenuation in the aorta lumen. The scan delay is calculated on the basis of CM arrival in the vessel and acquisition initiation. This increases efficiency of the angiographic phase (mean between aorta attenuation/CM dose). During the first pass of the CM bolus, there is maximum opacification of the aorta and its branches. In this phase, the true lumen is more intensely opacified, enabling differentiation from the false lumen in dissections. This phase is followed by a late-phase acquisition performed with a delay of around 80 s, which is useful for demonstrating possible CM extravasation in the case of wall rupture. In aortic dissections, the true lumen and false lumen will have the same level of opacification as a result of CM recirculation and homogeneous mixing with blood in the false lumen.

Multidetector-row Computed Tomography in Aortic Dissections

The clinical question asked of any diagnostic test in a patient with suspected aortic dissection is to identify the intimal flap and assess involvement of the ascending aorta: transoesophageal echocardiography (TOE), CT and MRI are all able to respond to this diagnostic enquiry [1,5].

In clinical practice, the main diagnostic tool used in aortic dissection is CT, which, according to some authors [6], has similar diagnostic accuracy as MRI and TOE: sensitivity of 100% for the three modalities; specificity of 100% for spiral

CT and 94% for TOE and MRI. MDCT has become the modality of choice for diagnosing aortic dissection, with sensitivity and specificity values close to 100%. Compared with MRI and, especially, TOE, CT can distinguish among the different thoracic and abdominal diseases included in the differential diagnosis [7,8], as it permits evaluation from the abdominal to the thoracic region or vice versa in very short examination times. CT provides a high level of accuracy and detail in acute dissection [9] and is able to solve many pulmonary, vascular and abdominal differential diagnoses, which justifies its use in preference to MRI [10]. The patient's clinical condition, the index of suspicion, the possibility of monitoring vital parameters, local situations related to technique accessibility and the different CT and MRI technology available, as well as experience in the use of these modalities, will affect and justify the choice of other methods [11–13].

MDCT allows panoramic, thin-section (1–3 mm) evaluation of the aorta within seconds. Although the key diagnostic clues are provided by CT angiography, the importance of preliminary unenhanced scans should not be overlooked. These scans can demonstrate endoluminal calcification, enlarged aorta, density differences between the two lumens and hyperdensity due to leaked or thrombosed blood in the wall, in periaortic regions, or in pleural and pericardiac effusions [14].

Distinction between the true and false lumen is fundamental both for surgical repair and for planning percutaneous treatment with an endovascular stent [15]. Before any treatment is undertaken, it is crucial to determine whether the major branches – i.e. the coronary, epiaortic, coeliac and mesenteric and renal arteries – originate from the true or false lumen, because the parenchymas and structures supplied by vesselsarising from the false lumen may become severely damaged when the false lumen is spontaneously or surgically occluded.

In acute forms, it is unlikely that a thrombus, which is prevalent in the false lumen will be detected. The differences in size between the two lumens do not depend on the false lumen compressing the true lumen but on the elastic retraction of the intima once it has lost adherence with the aortic wall. The most specific, albeit inconstant [16], radiological sign for distinguishing the true from the false lumen is the direct continuity between the true lumen of the dissected portion and the lumen of the uninvolved aorta proximal or distal to the dissection [16,17]. Demonstration of the intimal flap is very accurate and precise on CT and MRI of the descending aorta; the detached intima is perpendicular to the scan plane, has limited movement, and it is ideally situated for recognition on axial images.

In the ascending aorta, the detached intima may be more or less obliquely oriented in the scan plane and has greater mobility the more proximal the dissection. Therefore, in the ascending and transverse aorta, where the dissected flap may be parallel to the scan plane, its direct visualisation is less constant and more haphazard. In addition, in the ascending aorta, the flapping movements of the dissection flap, which can go from one wall to the other between a systole and a diastole, can misleadingly duplicate or triplicate the images of the intimal flap.

TEE in Aortic Disease

TEE is readily available in most institutions. The reported diagnostic sensitivities and specificities are comparable to those of the traditional "gold standards." Consequently, TEE has become increasingly popular as an imaging technique for suspected intrathoracic aortic dissection. Several authors have recently advocated the use of TEE as the sole diagnostic modality in suspected thoracic aortic dissection. TEE can be used as an

- Excellent tool for aortic valve diagnosis - Aortic insufficiency? Aortic Stenosis?
- Examination of other valves
- Excellent tool for reconstructive valve surgery
- Additional tool in aortic dissection in the operating room

Furthermore, Three-dimensional echocardiography is an emerging technique with tremendous potential in patients with aortic valve and ascending aortic pathologies.

Conclusion

Because patients with acute thoracic aortic syndrome are generally in critical condition and potentially requiring immediate surgery, it is mandatory for emergency departments to be equipped with high-performance diagnostic tools. The advent of multidetector spiral CT technology offers patients with suspected acute aortic disease the possibility of having a complete evaluation of the entire aorta in a single, very fast acquisition. It allows accurate visualisation of, for example, intimal dissections, associated pseudoaneurysms, involvement of secondary branches, extension to the aortic root and possible communications between true and false lumen.

Supplementing TEE findings with additional imaging studies may improve its diagnostic accuracy, especially in cases where TEE findings are only considered "probable" or when the imaging results are negative, but dissection is strongly suspected clinically. However, due to the rapid nature of the disease, time and the opportunity to save the patient may be lost while awaiting additional tests. Therefore, the treating physician must have a sound knowledge about the strengths and weaknesses of all available imaging tests. Such knowledge enables the physician to efficiently plan for diagnostic studies and incorporate the results into the patient's clinical picture to initiate effective and practical treatment.

References

1. Bonomo L, Di Fabio F, Rita Larici A, et al (2002) Non-traumatic thoracic emergencies: acute chest pain: diagnostic strategies. Eur Radiol 12:1872–1875
2. Jacquier A, Chabbert V, Vidal V, et al (2004) Imaging of the thoracic aorta in adults: when, how and why? J Radiol 85:854–869

3. Novelline RA, Rhea JT, Rao PM, et al (1999) Helical CT in emergency radiology. Radiology 213:321–339
4. Willoteaux S, Lions C, Gaxotte V, et al (2004) Imaging of aortic dissection by helical computed tomography (CT). Eur Radiol 14:1999–2008
5. Willens HJ, Kessler KM (1999) Transesophageal echocardiography in the diagnosis of diseases of the thoracic aorta. Part 1. Aortic dissection, aortic intramural hematoma, and penetrating atherosclerotic ulcer of the aorta. Chest 116:1772–1779
6. Sommer T, Fehske W, Holzknecht N, et al (1996) Aortic dissection: a comparative study of diagnosis with spiral CT, multiplanar transesophageal echocardiography, and MR imaging. Radiology 199:347–352
7. Costello P, Ecker CP, Tello R et al (1992) Assessment of the thoracic aorta by spiral CT. AJR Am J Roentgenol 158:1127–1130
8. Thoongsuwan N, Stern EJ (2002) Chest CT scanning for clinical suspected thoracic aortic dissection: beware the alternate diagnosis. Emerg Radiol 9:257–261
9. Zeman RK, Berman PM, Silverman PM, et al (1995) Diagnosis of aortic dissection: value of helical CT with multiplanar reformation and threedimensional rendering. AJR Am J Roentgenol 164:1375–1380
10. Rubin GD (2003) CT angiography of the thoracic aorta. Semin Roentgenol 38:115–134
11. Kobayashi Y, Ichikawa T, Matuura K, et al (1994) Efficacy of helical CT in the assessment of aortic disease. AJR Am J Roentgenol 162:56–57
12. Small JH, Dixon AK, Coulden RA, et al (1996) Fast CT for aortic dissection. Br J Radiol 69:900–905
13. Sebastià C, Pallisa E, Quirtoga S, et al (1999) Aortic dissection: diagnosis and follow-up with helical CT. Radiographics 19:45–60
14. Dore R, Preda L, Di Giulio G, et al (2000) Le urgenze toraciche cardiovascolari. Radiol Med 99:S117–S128
15. Lee DY, Williams DM, Abrams GD (1997) The dissected aorta. Part II. Differentiation of the true from the false lumen with intravascular US. Radiology 203:32–36
16. LePage M, Quint LE, Sonnad SS, et al (2001) Aortic dissection: CT features that distinguish true from false lumen. AJR Am J Roentgenol 177:207–211
17. Williams DM, Joshi A, Dake MD, et al (1994) Aortic cobwebs: an anatomic marker identifying the false lumen in aortic dissection - imaging and pathologic correlation. Radiology 190:167–174

Noninvasive Diagnosis of the Artery of Adamkiewicz

Kunihiro Yoshioka, Ryoichi Tanaka, and Shigeru Ehara

Summary It is important to assess the artery of Adamkiewicz before repair of the thoracoabdominal aorta. Several studies have demonstrated the feasibility and advantages of noninvasive assessment of the artery of Adamkiewicz with MR angiography and CT angiography. Recent advanced in MR and CT angiography have led to changes in the detectability of this artery. In our experience, CT and/or MR angiography are comparable or superior to conventional angiography in the evaluation of the artery of Adamkiewicz. CT and MR angiography can also diagnose the various types of the collateral circulations. MR angiography is superior for depiction of the artery of Adamkiewicz, especially when it arises from the false lumen of a dissecting aneurysm. CT angiography has a wide field of view and allows depiction of significant collateral pathways associated with internal thoracic artery and intercostals arteries. For the identification of the artery of Adamkiewicz, it is very important to distinguish between the artery and a vein.

Keywords Adamkiewicz artery · Spinal artery · Aortic aneurysm · Computed tomography (CT) · Magnetic resonance imaging (MRI)

Introduction

It is very important to identify the artery of Adamkiewicz in patients with thoracoabdominal or descending thoracic aortic aneurysms in order to minimize the risk of postoperative spinal cord ischemia and paraplegia. Although several investigators have attempted to depict the artery of Adamkiewicz preoperatively, the rate of postoperative paraplegia or paraparesis remains high, in the range of 5% to 10% (1–3). These critical complications are caused by ischemia in the territory supplied by the anterior spinal

K. Yoshioka, R. Tanaka, and S. Ehara
Department Radiology, Memorial Heart Center, Iwate Medical University

K. Yoshioka (✉)
19-1 Uchimaru, Morioka, Iwate 020-8505, Japan
e-mail: kyoshi@iwate-med.ac.jp

artery. In the thoracoabdominal region, the spinal cord is supplied by the great anterior radiculomedullary artery which is also known as the artery of Adamkiewicz. The artery of Adamkiewicz is a critical vessel that may supply the lower third of the spinal cord. It arises from the left intercostal or lumbar arteries in 68% to 73% of patients and at the level of 9th to 12th intercostal arteries in 62% to 75% of patients.

Anatomy and Imaging

It is also important to understand the entire anatomical course of the artery of Adamkiewicz. An intercostal artery or lumbar artery arising from the descending aorta divides into anterior and posterior branches. The posterior branch then subdivides into the radiculomedullary artery, the muscular branch, and the dorsal somatic branch. The radiculomedullary artery further subdivides into the anterior and posterior radiculomedullary arteries. The most dominant anterior radiculomedullary artery, with a diameter of 0.8 to 1.3mm, is called the artery of Adamkiewicz, which shows a characteristic hairpin turn configuration.

Recent studies with conventional selective angiography for the evaluation of the artery of Adamkiewicz have shown that the depiction rate ranges 43% to 86% (4–6). Although conventional angiography could achieve a higher depiction rate, severe critical complications occurred in 2% (5). This is unacceptable in the clinical setting. This is why we are looking forward to noninvasive diagnostic methods such as multidetector-row computed tomographic (CT) angiography and magnetic resonance (MR) angiography to evaluate the artery of Adamkiewicz.

Noninvasive assessment methods employing multidetector-row CT angiography (7,8) and MR angiography (8–10) have recently been introduced. In the several years since MR angiography and CT angiography were first employed to depict the artery of Adamkiewicz, these modalities have undergone substantial development.

Diagnosis

CT angiography using multiplanar reformation (MPR) and curved planar reformation (CPR) images can depict the artery of Adamkiewicz in a manner similar to conventional angiography. Based on clinical experience, it has been found that there is some variation in the hairpin turn configuration. In addition, the morphologic features of the anterior radiculomedullary vein and the artery are similar. It is therefore important to distinguish between the anterior radiculomedullary artery and the vein. The anterior spinal artery is small in caliber and follows a straight course, while the anterior spinal vein is larger and follows a more tortuous course than the artery. Based on embryological development, the length of ascent of the artery of Adamkiewicz is less than two to two and a half vertebral bodies in length. But It is sometimes difficult to distinguish between these two vessels on the basis of characteristic shape in the clinical setting.

Diagnosis of the Artery of Adamkiewicz

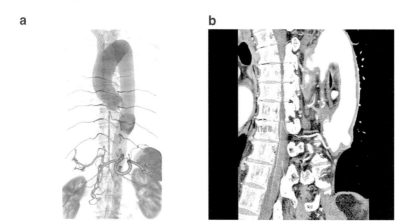

Fig. 1 Demonstration of the artery of Adamkiewicz by CT angiography. 74-year-old man with TAA. (**a**) Three-dimensional volume-rendered (VR) image, displayed with a semitransparent aorta and skeletal system, shows the artery of Adamkiewicz with hairpin turn configuration at the level of 10th thoracic vertebra. (**b**) Curved planar reformatted (CPR) image shows entire continuity between the aorta and the anterior spinal artery via the artery of Adamkiewicz

Our recommendation is to distinguish between these vessels based on the anatomical connection, i.e., to identify "continuity" between the aorta and the anterior spinal artery. The definitive diagnosis of such continuity is based on the depiction of a continuous vascular route involving the anterior spinal artery, the artery of Adamkiewicz, the radiculomedullary artery, the posterior branch of the intercostal artery, the intercostal artery, and the aorta, traced in the retrograde direction in CPR images (Fig. 1). The branching level of the artery of Adamkiewicz is determined on the basis of the anatomic level of the intercostal or lumbar artery from which the artery of Adamkiewicz is seen to arise. In turn, the anatomic level of the intercostal artery is defined as the level of the rib below which the artery runs. The use of volume-rendered (VR) images makes it possible to understand such continuity easily (11,12).

MR angiography can also clearly depict the continuity of the artery of Adamkiewicz with the use of CPR and VR images.

Imaging Techniques

CT Angiography

CT angiography was performed using a 64-channel multidetector-row helical CT scanner (Aquilion 64, Toshiba, Tokyo, Japan). The scanning parameters were as follows: 120 kV, 400 mA, 0.5-mm section thickness × 64 slices, 41.0 pitch, and 0.75-sec rotation speed. Scanning was performed from the 7th thoracic vertebra to the 2nd lumbar vertebra (with the appropriate scan range determined from a scout digital radiograph). A 20-gauge plastic intravenous catheter was placed in an antecubital vein and connected to a power injector (Autoenhance A-250, Nemoto Kyorindo, Tokyo, Japan). A total of 2.0 mL/kg body weight of high-osmolarity iopamidol (Iopamiron, Schering, Berlin, Germany; 370 mgI/mL) was administered at a rate of 3.5 mL/sec using the power injector, followed by a 35-mL normal saline flush, which was also injected at 3.5 mL/sec. The scan delay was set using an automatic scan triggering system (SureStart, Toshiba). A Zio M900 (Zio Software, Tokyo, Japan) was used to reconstruct the acquired data.

MR Angiography

MR angiography was performed using a 1.5-T superconducting MR imaging system (Signa EXCITE X1, GE Medical Systems, Milwaukee, WI) with system software 11.0 combined with a four-channel phased-array coil. The pulse sequence employed was a three-dimensional fast spoiled gradient-echo sequence with a chemical shift-selective fat suppression technique. The imaging parameters were as follows: 50- to 60-mm section thickness with 50–60 partitions (1-mm partition thickness), 0.5-mm reconstruction interval with the zero filling interpolation technique, 18-msec repetition time, 2.1-msec echo time, 40° flip angle, 32-Hz acquisition bandwidth, 168 × 240-mm field of view, 384 × 512 matrix, and 0.47 × 0.44-mm pixel size. The section orientation was sagittal, allowing coverage of the region from the 7th thoracic vertebra to the 2nd lumbar vertebra. The acquisition time was 4–6 minutes. A total of 0.2 mmol/kg body weight of gadopentetate dimeglumine (Gd-DTPA; Magnevist, Schering) was administered at a rate of 0.2 mL/sec using a power injector (Sonicshot 50, Nemoto Kyorindo), followed by a 20-mL normal saline flush, which was injected at 0.3 mL/sec. Injection was started 60–70 sec before the half-acquisition time. The Zio workstation was also used for reconstruction.

Collateral Circulation

In some cases of thoracoabdominal aortic aneurysm and dissecting aortic aneurysm, the surgeons observed ostial occlusion of the intercostal or lumbar arteries. By using the noninvasive methods described above, we were able to depict the presence of collaterals supplying the artery of Adamkiewicz. Many types of collaterals can be demonstrated by both MR angiography and CT angiography. The most common collateral vessel is muscular branch, and some connected to the distal portion of the intercostal arteries (13, 14). In one rare but important case, the left internal thoracic artery supplied the collateral circulation (15).

Based on our experience (13), the collaterals were observed supplied in 7 of 30 cases (23%), which indicates that this is not an uncommon finding.

Limitations of MR Angiography and CT Angiography

It is well known that osseous structures can sometimes interfere with the visualization of arteries. CT angiography has a number of disadvantages in the depiction of the artery of Adamkiewicz. Even when the bony structures are normal, it may be difficult to visualize an artery that runs close to the bony structures. CT angiography suffers from another limitation in patients with dissecting aneurysms. It is difficult to depict the artery of Adamkiewicz when the intercostal artery arises from the false lumen.

MR angiography suffers from a limited field of view (FOV) in sagittal imaging, and it is difficult to depict a collateral when it runs out of the FOV.

The reported detection rates have varied, but we recommend the combined use of both procedures, which provides detection rates of 97% for the hairpin turn configuration and 90% for the depiction of continuity (Table 1–3).

Table 1 Detection rates by CT angiography

Author	Year	"hairpin turn"	"continuity"
1) Takase K, et al (4-channel, slice thickness = 2 mm)	2002	90%	29%
2) Yoshioka K, et al (4-channel, slice thickness = 1 mm)	2003	80%	50%
3) Yoshioka K, et al (16-channel, slice thickness = 0.5 mm)	2006	83%	60%

1) Radiology 223: 39–45, 2002
2) Radiographics 23: 1215–1225, 2003
3) Radiographics 26: S63–S73, 2006

Table 2 Detection rates by MR angiography

Author	Year	"hairpin turn"	"continuity"
1) Yamada N et al.	2000	69%	NA*
2) Yoshioka K et al.	2003	67%	57%
3) Hyodoh H et al.	2005	84%	NA*
4) Yoshioka K et al.	2006	93%	80%
5) Nijenhuis RJ et al.	2007	100%	NA*

*NA: not available
1) J Comput Assist Tomogr 24: 362–368, 2000
2) Radiographics 23: 1215–1225, 2003
3) Radiology 236: 1004–1009, 2005
4) Radiographics 26: S63–S73, 2006
5) J Vasc Surg 45: 71–78, 2007

Table 3 Detection rates with the combination of CT and MR angiography

Author	Year	"hairpin turn"	"continuity"
1) Yoshioka K et al.	2003	90%	63%
2) Yoshioka K et al.	2006	97%	90%

1) Radiographics 23: 1215–1225, 2003
2) Radiographics 26: S63–S73, 2006

Conclusion

Noninvasive CT angiography and MR angiography are comparable or superior to conventional angiography in the evaluation of the artery of Adamkiewicz. We must emphasize the importance of correctly distinguishing between the artery of Adamkiewicz and the anterior radiculomedullary vein to ensure the safety in thoracoabdominal aortic repair.

References

1. Coselli JS, LeMaire SA, Miller CC 3rd, et al (2000) Mortality and paraplegia after thoracoabdominal aortic aneurysm repair: a risk factor analysis. Ann Thorac Surg 69: 409–414.
2. Estrera AL, Miller CC 3rd, Huynh TT, et al (2001) Neurologic outcome after thoracic and thoracoabdominal aortic aneurysm repair. Ann Thorac Surg 72: 1225–1231.
3. Cambria RP, Clouse WD, Davison JK, et al (2002) Thoracoabdominal aneurysm repair: results with 337 operations performed over a 15-year interval. Ann Surg 236: 471–479.
4. Heinemann MK, Brassel F, Herzog T, et al (1998) The role of spinal angiography in operations on the thoracic aorta: myth or reality? Ann Thorac Surg 65: 346–351.
5. Kieffer E, Fukui S, Chiras J, et al (2002) Spinal cord arteriography: a safe adjunct before descending thoracic or thoracoabdominal aortic aneurysmectomy. J Vasc Surg 35: 262–268.
6. Williams GM, Roseborough GS, Thomas HW, et al (2004) Preoperative selective intercostals angiography in patients undergoing thoracoabdominal aneurysm repair. J Vasc Surg 39: 314–320.
7. Yoshioka K, Niinuma H, Ohira A, et al (2003) MR angiography and CT angiography of the artery of Adamkiewicz: noninvasive preoperative assessment of thoracoabdominal aortic aneurysm. Radiographics 23: 1215–1225.
8. Takase K, Sawamura Y, Igarashi K, et al (2002) Demonstration of the artery of Adamkiewicz at multi-detector row helical CT. Radiology 223: 39–45.
9. Yamada N, Takamiya M, Kuribayashi S, et al (2000) MRA of the Adamkiewicz artery: a preoperative study for thoracic aortic aneurysm. J Comput Assist Tomogr 24: 362–368.
10. Hyodoh H, Kawaharada N, Akiba H, et al (2005) Usefulness of preoperative detection of artery of Adamkiewicz with dynamic contrast-enhanced MR angiography. Radiology 236: 1004–1009.
11. Yoshioka K, Niinuma H, Kawakami T, et al (20005) Three-dimensional demonstration of the artery of Adamkiewicz with contrast-enhanced magnetic resonance angiography. Ann Thorac Surg 79: 1785.
12. Yoshioka K, Niinuma H, Ohira A, et al (2004) Three-dimensional demonstration of the artery of Adamkiewicz by multidetector-row computed tomography. Ann Thorac Surg 78: 719.
13. Yoshioka K, Niinuma H, Ehara S, et al (2006) MR angiography and CT angiography of the artery of Adamkiewicz: state of the art. Radiographics 26: S63–73.
14. Yoshioka K, Niinuma H, Ogino Y, et al (2006) Three-dimensional demonstration of the collateral circulation to the artery of Adamkiewicz with 16-row multislice computed tomography. Ann Thorac Surg 81: 749.
15. Yoshioka K, Niinuma H, Kawazoe K, et al (2005) Three-dimensional demonstration of the collateral circulation to the artery of Adamkiewicz via internal thoracic artery with 16-row multi-slice CT. Eur J Cardiothorac Surg 28: 492.

Lecture 2
Novel Technologies in Diagnosis and Treatment for Aortic Diseases

Gene Analysis of Marfan Syndrome

Naomichi Matsumoto

Abstract Marfan syndrome (MFS, OMIM #154700) is an autosomal dominant connective tissue disorder, clinically presenting with cardinal features of skeletal, ocular, and cardiovascular systems. In a classical concept of MFS, changes in connective tissue integrity can be explained by defects in fibrillin-1, a major component of extracellular microfibrils. Recently *TGFBR2* and *TGFBR1* mutations were identified in a subset of patients with MFS (MFS2, OMIM #154705) and other MFS-related disorders including Loeys-Dietz syndrome (LDS, #OMIM 609192) and familial thoracic aortic aneurysms and dissections (TAAD2, #OMIM 608987) [1]. These data may indicate that genetic heterogeneity exists in MFS and its related conditions and regulation of TGF-β signaling plays a significant role in these disorders. It is noteworthy that losartan, an angiotensin II type 1 receptor (AT1) antagonist, has been highlighted as a potential drug for protection of aortic aneurysm in a mice MFS model through suppression of abnormal TGF-β upregulation. In this lecture, comprehensive genetic study of MFS and MFS-related disorder in Japan is presented. Furthermore future direction for genetic study of a more common disorder, aortic dissection will be discussed.

Keywords Marfan syndrome · *FBN1* · *TGFBR2* · *TGFBR1* · Loeys-Dietz syndrome

Introduction

Marfan syndrome (MFS, OMIM #154700) is a connective tissue disorder with autosomal dominant inheritance. MFS is clinically diagnosed according to the Ghent criteria, which describe pleiotropic manifestations affecting multiple

---

N. Matsumoto (✉)
Department of Human Genetics, Yokohama City University Graduate School of Medicine, Fukuura 3-9, Kanazawa-ku, Yokohama 236-0004, Japan
e-mail: naomat@yokohama-cu.ac.jp

organs [2]. Cardiovascular symptoms could be one of important determinants for lives in MFS patients. Aortic root dilatation and dissection of the ascending aorta are major criteria, while mitral valve prolapse, dilatation of the pulmonary artery, calcified mitral annuls at younger that 40 years, and other dilatation of dissection of aorta are minor criteria.

Recent Understanding of Genes Responsible for MFS and MFS-related Disorders

Since the first discovery of *FBN1* mutation at 15q21.1 [3], more than 600 *FBN1* mutations are registered in the UMD-*FBN1* database for MFS and its associated disorders (http://www.umd.be:2030/) [4]. The mutation detection rate of *FBN1* in MFS varies among studies, ranging from 9 to 91% [5–7], implicating that missing mutations by each analytical method or genetic heterogeneity in MFS. In 2004, patients with MFS2 (OMIM #154705) linked to 3p24.1 were shown to have mutations in the *TGFBR2* gene, encoding the transmembrane receptor type II of TGFβ [8]. Subsequently *TGFBR2* and *TGFBR1* mutations were identified in Loeys-Dietz syndrome (LDS, OMIM #609192) [9]. LDS is characterized by hypertelorism, bifid uvula, cleft palate, generalized arterial tortuosity, ascending aortic aneurysm and dissection. Furthermore *TGFBR2* mutations were found in familial thoracic aortic aneurysms and dissections (TAAD) [10] as well as Shprintzen-Goldberg craniosynostosis syndrome (SGS, OMIM #182212) [11].

Japanese Cohort Study

Comprehensive genetic analysis of Japanese MFS and MFS-related conditions was performed in our laboratory [12, 13]. A total of 107 MFS-related patients were recruited: 81 MFS and MFS-suspected patients, 16 Beals syndrome (BS, OMIM #121050) patients, and 10 LDS-suspected patients. BS which is caused by *FBN2* mutations [14] is also included in our study, presenting with skeletal features including arachnodactyly, dolichostenomelia, scoliosis and pectus deformity basically without cardiovasucular or ocular features. *FBN1*, *FBN2*, *TGFBR1* and *TGFBR2* were analyzed by direct sequencing of exon-based PCR. Mutations of *FBN1*, *TGFBR1*, and *TGFBR2* were found in 45 (56%), 1 (1.2%), and 2 (2.5%) out of 81 MFS/MFS-suspected patients. *FBN2* were mutated in 4 (25%) of 16 BS patients, but no *TGFBR1* or *TGFBR2* abnormality was identified in BS. Regarding LDS, only 5 *TGFBR2* mutations (50%) were found in 5 of 10 patients.

MFS2 and LDS

Whether an MFS2 phenotype exists as a separate disorder from LDS is debatable. *TGFBR1* and *TGFBR2* aberrations are highly prevalent in LDS and their mutations are rare (1–2%) in MFS as indicated in our study. Although the original MFS2 patients with *TGFBR2* mutations [8] could not be reasonably reevaluated for the presence of LDS features such as bifid uvula, hypertelorism, craniosynostosis, and arterial tortuosity, at least three reports have since described *TGFBR1* or *TGFBR2* mutations in classic MFS patients in whom LDS was ruled out [15–17]. It should be noted that arterial tortuosity, a defining feature of LDS, was not systematically evaluated in any of the four studies [12, 15–17]. Moreover, two research groups were unable to identify *TGFBR2* mutations in twenty-nine MFS patients (*FBN1* was normal in 24 and unknown in five) [18] and in 7 patients (*FBN1* was normal) with MFS compatible with the Ghent criteria [9]. Thus, the question of whether an MFS2 phenotype and LDS should be classified as the same disorder remains to be solved. However, it is obvious that recognition of LDS phenotype in patients leads to the higher mutation detection rate of *TGFBRs*.

Abnormal TGF-β Signaling in MFS

A recent study revealed that LTBP-1 [one of latent TGF-β biding proteins (LTBPs)] and fibrillin interact in vitro and suggested that fibrillin-1 may stabilize the latent TGF-β complexes in the extracellular matrix (ECM) [19]. Three strains of transgenic mice, each harboring a different type of *Fbn1* mutation, displayed several MFS features with variable severity [20–22]. Increased TGFβ activity was observed in at least four organs (lung, mitral valve, aortic and dural tissues), possibly as a result of excess free large latency complex due to inadequate stabilization within the ECM. Administration of an anti-TGFβ neutralizing antibody rescued the lung, mitral valve, and aortic tissue phenotypes in mice [23–25]. Furthermore, aortic aneurysm was prevented by the administration of losartan, an angiotensin II type 1 receptor blocker that alleviates increased TGF-β activity in mouse models [23]. Thus even in human, losartan may be expected to prevent aortic aneurysm in MFS.

Genetic Study for Aortic Dissection

Finally, genetic study of aortic dissection is discussed. In the annual report of the Japanese association for thoracic surgery, about 4125 cases of dissecting aneurysms were surgically operated in 2005 [26]. It is known that most cases are not associated with apparent genetic disorders such as MFS and Ehlers-Danlos syndrome. Two strategies for study of aortic dissection are proposed. Re-sequencing strategy of genes responsible for genetic disorders presenting with aortic dissection according to the model of multiple rare variants leading to aortic dissection. The other is the whole genome SNP association study according to common variants resulting in aortic dissection. Re-sequencing chip is now being designed in our laboratory. Both strategies may hopefully open new understanding of the common form of aortic dissections which could lead to its prevention and therapy.

Acknowledgements Patients and their families, all the collaborating doctors, and the Marfan Net Work Japan are highly appreciated for participating in this study. Grants were supported by CREST, JST; Takeda Science Foundation, and Uehara Memorial Foundation.

References

1. Mizuguchi T and Matsumoto N (2007) Recent progress in genetics of Marfan syndrome and Marfan-associated disorders. J Hum Genet 52:1–12
2. De Paepe A, Devereux RB, Dietz HC, et al (1996) Revised diagnostic criteria for the Marfan syndrome. Am J Med Genet 62:417–426
3. Dietz HC, Cutting GR, Pyeritz RE, et al (1991) Marfan syndrome caused by a recurrent de novo missense mutation in the fibrillin gene. Nature 352:337–339
4. Collod-Beroud G, Le Bourdelles S, Ades L, et al (2003) Update of the UMD-FBN1 mutation database and creation of an FBN1 polymorphism database. Hum Mutat. 22:199–208
5. Katzke S, Booms P, Tiecke F, et al (2002) TGGE screening of the entire FBN1 coding sequence in 126 individuals with marfan syndrome and related fibrillinopathies. Hum Mutat 20:197–208
6. Loeys B, De Backer J, Van Acker P, et al (2004) Comprehensive molecular screening of the FBN1 gene favors locus homogeneity of classical Marfan syndrome. Hum Mutat 24:140–146
7. Tynan K, Comeau K, Pearson M, et al (1993) Mutation screening of complete fibrillin-1 coding sequence: report of five new mutations, including two in 8-cysteine domains. Hum Mol Genet 2:1813–1821
8. Mizuguchi T, Collod-Beroud G, Akiyama T, et al (2004) Heterozygous TGFBR2 mutations in Marfan syndrome. Nat Genet 36:855–860
9. Loeys BL, Chen J, Neptune ER, et al (2005) A syndrome of altered cardiovascular, craniofacial, neurocognitive and skeletal development caused by mutations in TGFBR1 or TGFBR2. Nat Genet 37:275–281
10. Pannu H, Fadulu V T, Chang J, et al (2005) Mutations in transforming growth factor-beta receptor type II cause familial thoracic aortic aneurysms and dissections. Circulation 112:513–520
11. Kosaki K, Takahashi D, Udaka T, et al (2006) Molecular pathology of Shprintzen-Goldberg syndrome. Am J Med Genet A 140:104–108; author reply 109–110
12. Sakai H, Visser R, Ikegawa S, et al (2006) Comprehensive genetic analysis of relevant four genes in 49 patients with Marfan syndrome or Marfan-related phenotypes. Am J Med Genet A 140:1719–1725
13. Nishimura A, Sakai H, Ikegawa S, et al (2007) FBN2, FBN1, TGFBR1, and TGFBR2 analyses in congenital contractural arachnodactyly. Am J Med Genet A 143:694–698
14. Putnam EA, Zhang H, Ramirez F, et al (1995) Fibrillin-2 (FBN2) mutations result in the Marfan-like disorder, congenital contractural arachnodactyly. Nat Genet 11:456–458
15. Disabella E, Grasso M, Marziliano N, et al (2006) Two novel and one known mutation of the TGFBR2 gene in Marfan syndrome not associated with FBN1 gene defects. Eur J Hum Genet 14:34–38

16. Matyas G, Arnold E, Carrel T, et al (2006) Identification and in silico analyses of novel TGFBR1 and TGFBR2 mutations in Marfan syndrome-related disorders. Hum Mutat 27: 760–769
17. Singh KK, Rommel K, Mishra A, et al (2006) TGFBR1 and TGFBR2 mutations in patients with features of Marfan syndrome and Loeys-Dietz syndrome. Hum Mutat 27:770–777
18. Ki CS, Jin DK, Chang SH, et al (2005) Identification of a novel TGFBR2 gene mutation in a Korean patient with Loeys-Dietz aortic aneurysm syndrome; no mutation in TGFBR2 gene in 30 patients with classic Marfan's syndrome. Clin Genet 68:561–563
19. Isogai Z, Ono RN, Ushiro S, et al (2003) Latent transforming growth factor beta-binding protein 1 interacts with fibrillin and is a microfibril-associated protein J Biol Chem 278:2750–2757
20. Judge DP, Biery NJ, Keene DR, et al (2004) Evidence for a critical contribution of haploinsufficiency in the complex pathogenesis of Marfan syndrome. J Clin Invest 114:172–181
21. Pereira L, Andrikopoulos K, Tian J, et al (1997) Targetting of the gene encoding fibrillin-1 recapitulates the vascular aspect of Marfan syndrome. Nat Genet 17:218–222
22. Pereira L, Lee SY, Gayraud B, et al (1999) Pathogenetic sequence for aneurysm revealed in mice underexpressing fibrillin-1. Proc Natl Acad Sci USA 96: 3819–3823
23. Habashi JP, Judge DP, Holm TM, et al (2006) Losartan, an AT1 antagonist, prevents aortic aneurysm in a mouse model of Marfan syndrome. Science 312:117–121
24. Neptune ER, Frischmeyer PA, Arking DE, et al (2003) Dysregulation of TGF-beta activation contributes to pathogenesis in Marfan syndrome. Nat Genet 33:407–411
25. Ng CM, Cheng A, Myers LA, et al (2004) TGF-beta-dependent pathogenesis of mitral valve prolapse in a mouse model of Marfan syndrome. J Clin Invest 114:1586–1592
26. Ueda Y, Osada H, Osugi H (2007) Thracic and cardiovascular surgery in Japan during 2005. Annual report by the Japanese Association for Thoracic Surgery. Gen Thorac Cardiovasc Surg 55:377–399

Evolving Medical Therapy for Abdominal Aortic Aneurysms

Rajdeep Deb, Hosaam H. Nasr, Ranjeet Brar, and Matthew M. Thompson

Summary Abdominal Aortic Aneurysms (AAAs) affect 5%–10% of men over 65 years. Ultrasound screening has been shown to reduce mortality. Its implementation will increase the incidence of newly diagnosed asymptomatic AAAs, but ninety percent of screen detected lesions are below current thresholds for elective surgical repair. The treatment option in these cases is either surveillance or conservative management.

AAA patients often have other associated risk-factors such as atherosclerosis, hypertension and a history of smoking all of which confer additional cardiovascular risk. 62% of AAA patients have one or more cardiac risk factors, and many deaths in the perioperative period are cardiac in origin. This realisation has lead to the evolution of medical, as well as surgical management of aneurysmal patients. Current medical management comprises cardiovascular risk reduction in all AAA patients, and perioperative optimisation in those undergoing surgical repair.

Research has demonstrated that simple biomechanical stress and shearing forces are not the only cause of aneurysm expansion and rupture. There is now greater understanding of the biological processes involved. As a result, new strategies have been suggested to modify aneurysmal growth, via manipulation of these processes. These will form the basis of future developments in medical management of aneurysmal disease.

Keywords aortic aneurysm · medical management · pathophysiology · pharmacotherapy · aneurysm expansion.

R. Deb, H.H. Nasr, R. Brar, and M.M. Thompson
St George's Vascular Institute, Department of Vascular Surgery, St Georges Hospital NHS Trust Blackshaw Road, London, SW17 0QT, UK

M.M. Thompson (✉)
St George's Vascular Institute, Department of Vascular Surgery, St Georges Hospital NHS Trust Blackshaw Road, London, SW17 0QT, UK
e-mail: Matt.Thompson@stgeorges.nhs.uk

Introduction

The prevalence of aneurysmal disease is increasing in the western world and in the UK currently accounts for 8000 deaths annually. Most aneurysm related deaths are as a result of rupture of previously undetected asymptomatic aneurysms, a diagnosis which carries an overall mortality of approximately 80% [1]. There are also significant cost implications for the local health service [2–3]. AAA screening has been shown to reduce mortality, as well as be cost-effective [2, 4–5] and has resulted in national and local ultrasound based programmes.

AAA's primarily affect middle aged and elderly male smokers, and as such there is an increased prevalence of atherosclerosis and other associated cardiovascular pathologies in this population [6]. The majority of patients undergoing vascular surgery have one or more cardiac risk factors, with 20% deemed high-risk as a result of significant stress induced ischemia [7]. AAA patients are at increased risk of fatal and non-fatal cardiovascular events in the pre and post-operative periods. Female AAA patients have twice the associated mortality as compared to their male counterparts [8–9].

In suitable patients the rationale for early elective surgical repair of large AAA's is clear [10–11], and open repair has been the mainstay of surgical management since the 1950's. Minimally invasive endovascular aneurysm repair (EVAR) is now an established alternative, and is associated with lower short-term mortality rates [12]. Long-term mortality figures however remained unchanged between the two operative methods. Endovascular repair is not suitable for all patients, being largely dependent on aneurysm morphology. 90% of screen detected AAA's are however below the current threshold for any surgical intervention [1, 6]. Since the natural history of small aneurysms is to expand and eventually rupture, ultrasound based surveillance is the primary intervention instigated, with a view to eventual repair once appropriate. Conservative treatment is applicable where repair would carry too high a risk of mortality or where it is unlikely to improve life expectancy.

In view of this and the high cardiovascular risk associated with aneurysmal disease the current role of medical management in AAA patients is to reduce cardiovascular risk factors, as well as patient optimisation in the perioperative period.

Current Medical Management

Cardiovascular Risk Reduction

In all patients, especially those deemed unfit for elective surgery, cardiovascular risk reduction is the mainstay of treatment. Modifiable risk factors include smoking and hypertension. Smoking is consistently associated with AAA expansion and rupture. The relative risk of AAA rupture is increased 4.6 fold in cigarette smokers, and 2.4 fold in pipe/cigar smokers. Smoking cessation advice should therefore be reinforced to every AAA patient. Hypertension has also been found to confer an increased risk of AAA rupture, with raised mean arterial or diastolic or diastolic pressure being more predictive of risk of rupture than systolic measurements [13–14]. In AAA patients ACE inhibitors should be in the first line therapy to control hypertension. Their effectiveness in reducing expansion and rupture rates in animal models of AAA was translated to a large retrospective population based case-control study which demonstrated clearly that their use in AAA patients reduced the incidence of rupture [15].

The beneficial role of HMG CoA Reductase inhibitors (statins) in coronary and cerebrovascular atherosclerosis is well established [16]. Statins have also been associated with reducing AAA growth and risk of rupture. This is thought to be a result of their inhibitory effects on matrix metalloproteinase's, key enzymes involved in AAA physiology [17]. Statin use is also indicated as a result of the effects on cardiovascular mortality. (see peri-operative management)

Arthrosclerosis and intra-luminal thrombus in AAA, have been identified as playing key role is AAA development [18]. Though there are no significant large scale studies looking specifically into their use in aneurysmal disease, antiplatelet therapy in the form of low dose aspirin or clopidogrel is indicated in view of their protective effects on the cardiovascular system.

Perioperative Medical Therapy

The medical optimisation of cardio-respiratory and renal function prior to elective aneurysm repair results in reduced postoperative organ dysfunction [19]. Medical management also has a role in the emergency setting, with permissive hypotensive resuscitation playing a key role in stabilisation of the ruptured AAA patient prior to surgery. With careful patient selection, the practice of hypotensive haemostasis has been shown to result in reduced patient mortality following emergency endovascular repair of ruptured AAA [6, 20–21].

The majority of perioperative mortality is related to cardiovascular causes. Beta-adrenergic receptor antagonists (beta-blockers) reduce heart rate and contractility, and consequently myocardial oxygen demand. They have been shown to reduce cardiac complications in patients with acute myocardial infarctions, silent ischemia and heart failure [7]. The hypothesis that perioperative beta-blockade of patients undergoing vascular surgery would improve cardiac outcome was evaluated by Poldermans et al [7] in a multi-centre, randomised trial. Death from cardiac causes, or non-fatal myocardial infarctions was reduced 10-fold in high risk patients undergoing vascular surgery when randomised to Bisoprolol as well as standard care. Similar results were not demonstrated using Atenolol or Metoprolol [22–23] though it has been suggested that this maybe be due the shorter duration of beta-blockade in these studies [24].

As well their effects on AAA growth and rupture rates, statins have been documented to reduce the risk of perioperative cardiovascular events. Kertai et al [25] found that long term use of statins led to a three-fold risk reduction in cardiovascular deaths following open elective AAA surgery. Review of the EUROSTAR registry, showed that use of statins in patients who underwent EVAR was associated with reduced overall mortality [26].

Future Medical Management

It is now clear that simple biomechanical stress and shearing forces are not the only cause of aneurysm expansion and rupture. Greater understandings of the biological processes involved have lead to the suggestion of new and novel pharmacotherapy for the modification of aneurysmal growth [13]. Current medical management has been shown to have some effects on aneurysm growth [6]. Ongoing work on animal models of aneurysms suggests that aneurysm regression may be possible, but whether this can be translated into human studies is unclear at present. The role of effective pharmacotherapy would be to slow the growth of small lesions and therefore reduce the need for surgery, to reduce rupture rates in those with large aneurysms denied surgery and to reduce aortic neck expansion following endovascular and conventional aneurysm repair. (See Fig. 1)

It has long been believed that AAA results from complications of atherosclerosis [27]. Although advanced aneurysmal disease may have characteristics

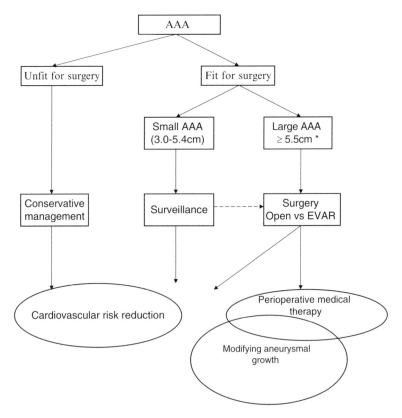

Fig. 1 Management of Abdominal Aortic Aneurysms. Abbreviations: AAA, Abdominal Aortic Aneurysm; EVAR, Endovascular Aneurysm Repair. *Or small aneurysm rapidly expanding/symptomatic

resembling atheroocclusive disease, aneurysmal lesions are associated with transmural architectural destruction caused by degredation of the arterial extracellular matrix. Many other pathophysiological processes have been implicated in AAA pathogenesis, expansion and rupture. These include apoptosis, adventitial and transmural inflammatory cell infiltration and angiogenesis [28–37]. Familial predisposition has been noted in AAA disease, whereby 15% of patients with AAA have a positive family history. A distinct gene locus has been mapped for the condition, compared to those identified for other aortic disease. Identification of the defective genes associated with the disease is essential for understanding the disease process.

Pathophysiology of AAA

Inflammation and Proteolysis

In AAA disease, the inflammatory response within aortic media and adventitia could be responsible for their eventual destruction. Inflammatory cell infiltrates, which include, B lymphocytes, T cells, mast cells, macrophages and dendritic cells are abundant in AAA tissue. This is thought to be a response to intimal damage caused by oxidised lipids. This inflammatory response could be intensified by further release of pro-inflammatory cytokines. IL-6 and interferon-γ were found to be significantly elevated in aneurysmal tissue compared with both atherosclerotic and normal control tissue [38]. Juvonen et al also demonstrated that in patients with underlying aneurysmal disease, there was a measurable elevation in circulating IL-6, IL-1β, TNF-α and INF-γ compared with coronary heart disease patients and normal controls [39]. Eventually, this inflammatory reaction will lead to extracellular protein matrix destruction by activating proteolytic digestion.

Extracellular proteins maintain the integrity and tensile strength of blood vessels. Under normal conditions, the extracellular protein matrix undergoes minimal degradation because of the balanced and controlled expression of proteolytic enzymes and their inhibitors. In the pathologic state this balance is disrupted by activation and over-expression of those proteolytic enzymes. The best studied group of such enzymes are matrix metalloproteinases (MMPs). The majority of MMPs are released by inflammatory cells, mainly macrophages. Other cells involved in MMP release are smooth muscle cells (SMCs), which produce MMP 9.

The loss of elastin and collagen, mediated by the proteolytic matrix metalloproteinases is thought to be responsible for aortic wall expansion and rupture [28]. With progressive loss of elastin, established AAAs are composed largely of collagen types I and III [27]. MMP 2 and MMP 9, which are both elastolytic and collagenolytic were found to be over-expressed in both human and experimental AAAs [40–42]. Other MMPs have also been implicated in the development of AAAs, such as MMP 1, MMP 3 and MMP 13 [43–45]. Further work showed that there was a localised increase in MMP 8 & 9 in the ruptured edge of human AAA tissue [46]. Tissue inhibitors of MMP (TIMP) have also been shown to play a role in preventing aneurysm rupture [47]. Since MMPs are known key players in angiogenesis, the pathological role of this process in aneurysm rupture was further investigated. Choke et al showed that there was increased medial neovascularisation and over-expression of pro-angiogenic cytokines in the rupture site of AAA compared to non-ruptured controls [48].

Another enzyme thought to play a pivotal role in extracellular matrix proteolysis is plasmin [49]. This proteolytic enzyme can exert its action on aneurysmal vessels by directly digesting the extracellular matrix, or indirectly, through activating zymogen (inactive) MMPs. Other serine proteases such as uPA and tPA have also been shown to be over-expressed in aneurysms compared to normal aortic tissue [43,49,50].

Infection and Autoimmunity

Infective organisms have been implicated in aneurysm formation. There are reports that up to 55% of aneurysms show evidence of Chlamydia pneumoniae infection. In an experimental model, aneurysm formation was induced by periodic application of C pneumoniae. Others have reported aneurysm development associated with salmonella infection [51–53].

It has been previously suggested that AAA disease develops secondary to an autoimmune response. This concept was supported by previous observations of lymphocytic and dendritic cell infiltration. Immunoglobulin G isolated from aneurysmal specimens has been shown to be immunoreactive with normal components of the aortic wall and with soluble proteins extracted from normal aortic tissue. Mutations at the HLA-DR locus, which have been implicated in other autoimmune disorders such as rheumatoid arthritis, were found to be associated with AAA disease [54].

Oxidative Stress

Oxidative stress is thought to play a major role in systemic arterial disease, including aneurysms. In aneurysmal tissue, the level of superoxides was found to be significantly high when compared to adjacent non-aneurysmal tissue, or healthy controls [55]. Elastase infusion into a rodent model significantly increased the expression of genes associated with oxidative stress and reduced expression of antioxidant genes [56]. In addition, products of oxidation have been found to be promoters of SMC apoptosis, MMP expression and activation. This clearly shows a correlation between oxidative stress and aneurysm formation and highlights the necessity to further investigate antioxidant agents as possible therapeutic modalities that could halt aneurysm formation and progression.

Genetic Factors in Aneurysm Disease

There is a clear genetic pattern in the occurrence of aneurysm disease. Approximately 15% of patients with AAA have a positive family history. Segregation analysis demonstrated a possibility that predisposition to AAA disease is determined by a recessive gene at a major autosomal diallelic locus [57,58]. The AAA loci are on chromosome 19q13 and 4q13 [59]. The evidence for genetic heterogeneity suggests that more loci have to be identified. This area of research will always pose a challenge for researchers, because of the level of complexity and the large number of patients needed.

Pharmacotherapy in AAA Management

Pharmacotherapy aims to decrease the expansion and rupture rate of aortic aneurysms by modifying aortic wall biology. Having identified the need for pharmacotherapeutic treatment of a large cohort of patients currently managed by surveillance and risk factor modification [1], it is worth summarising the ideal properties such an agent requires for effective application.

A common feature of the complexity of biologically evolved systems, that we have alluded to above, is redundancy of biological pathways [60]. Aneurysms clearly develop as a consequence of multiple mechanistic pathways and an agent that antagonises any single pathway is likely to prove ineffective. An effective agent must therefore be pleiotropic, exerting 'many actions' on pathogenic processes. Further, it must prove its efficacy by means of large scale clinical trials. As we envisage it would be necessary to remain on lifelong treatment, the drug must have an excellent safety profile. Several putative agents have been identified and clinical trials undertaken.

β-blockade

Early animal studies, in the broad-breasted white turkey [61], showed β-blockade with propanolol to retard aneurysm development. This effect was not attributable to blood pressure control, but seemed a distinct biological mechanism. Aortic tensile strength was found to be increased after treatment, due to induction of lysyl oxidase, which promoted stable cross-linkage between elastin fibrils, and retarded cross-linkage between collagen molecules (increasing collagen cross-linkage is a feature of ageing). Results were not fully reproducible in mouse models [62], however interest was sufficient to initiate a human randomised controlled trial (RCT) of Propranolol, and results were reported in 2002 [63]. 548 Patients were recruited to this high quality multicentre prospective RCT, randomised to propanolol treatment or placebo arms. They were then followed with serial 6-monthly abdominal ultrasound scans for a median of

2.5 years. No significant difference was found in either aneurysm expansion or death rates between placebo and propanolol groups, but the latter reported a high incidence of side effects, poorer quality of life and were more likely to discontinue medication and withdraw from the trial. Subsequent interest in Propranolol has been subdued.

NSAIDS

The central role of inflammation in aneurysm pathogenesis has led to attempts to modify these in animal models using cyclosporin, methylprednisolone [64], and TNF-BP (tumour necrosis factor antagonist) [65] with a measure of success. While the high degree of immunosuppression thus engendered is inappropriate for patient use, results indicated the potential benefits of non-steroidal anti-inflammatory (NSAID) drugs.

Indomethacin, a non selective cyclo-oxygenase inhibitor, has been shown to reduce expression of MMP-9 in rats [66], and though MMP-9 was not down-regulated in human aortic tissue ex-vivo samples, expression of the pro-inflammatory cytokines IL1-β, IL6, and PGE_2 was reduced [67]. Interestingly, recent analysis of a 'UK small aneurysm trial' patient sub-set, taking Indomethacin during the study, has shown it to inhibit aneurysm growth in-vivo [68]. Gastric, renal and hepatic side effects remain the major setback for prolonged NSAID use.

'Antibiotics' as MMP Inhibitors

Both the tetracyclines (Doxycycline) and macrolides (Roxithromycin, Azithromycin) have been shown to decrease MMP-9 activity [69]. Doxycycline is also the treatment antibiotic of choice for chlamydial infection, which has also been implicated in the pathogenesis of both aneurysmal and peripheral vascular disease [70,71].

A number of small clinical RCTs have been conducted [72–4] however promising results were tempered by small size of the trials and limited follow up period. More extensive trials are required to fully evaluate the efficacy of these drugs.

Although more specific MMP inhibitors have been developed, particularly in the field of oncology [75], problems of stability and toxicity have thus far prevented their introduction into clinical trials.

HMG Co-A Reductase Inhibitors (Statins)

Statins have pleiotropic actions that could modify biochemical activities implicated in aneurysm pathogenesis. Significant reduction was observed in both in-vitro [76] and in-vivo macrophage and smooth muscle cell expression of MMP-9 and MMP-3 in human aortic tissue [16]. They also decrease transcription of pro inflammatory cytokines, thus exerting a well described anti-inflammatory effect [77]. The clear benefits in reducing both cardiac events and peripheral atherosclerosis are described above [25].

Ultrasonographic surveillance studies of small AAAs have shown statin use to halve AAA expansion rates [78], while a small RCT demonstrated reduction of tissue MMP-9 by 40% in patients taking statins compared with those taking a placebo prior to elective open surgical repair [17]. This latter trial had to close early due to increasing statin use among eligible patients, but even with small numbers, the results were significant. Further large scale trials have been virtually precluded by the overwhelming evidence supporting increasing use of statins.

Peroxisome Proliferator-Activated Receptor γ

Thiazolodine-diones (rosiglitazone, pioglitazone) have recently been shown to inhibit vascular endothelial growth factor-induced angiogenesis; neo-angiogenesis has been implicated in aneurysm development and rupture. They also exert an anti-inflammatory action via reduced transcription of IL-6 and adhesion molecules. Collagen and extracellular matrix production is also up-regulated, while MMP-9 is down-regulated. This is thought to occur via the inhibition of phosphorylation and thus inhibition of activation of the MAPK signal transduction cascade (NFκβ, ERK).

Evolving Medical Management for AAA

While great strides have been made in understanding aneurysm pathogenesis at the molecular level, further elucidation of mechanisms will undoubtedly facilitate the expanding field of medical management for small aneurysms. The most effective agents are those with pleiotropic actions. Statins are probably effective in this regard as well as being well tolerated. Other agents acting on signal transduction mechanisms are promising avenues for ongoing and future research.

References

1. Thompson MM (2003) Controlling the expansion of Abdominal Aortic Aneurysms. Br J Surg 90: 897–898
2. Ashton HA, Buxton MJ, Day NE, et al (2002) Multicentre Aneurysm Screening Study Group. The Multicentre Aneurysm Screening Study (MASS) into the effect of abdominal aortic aneurysm screening on mortality in men: a randomised controlled trial. Lancet 360:1531–1539
3. Tang T, Lindop M, Munday I, et al (2003) A cost analysis of surgery for ruptured abdominal aortic aneurysm. Eur J Vasc Endovasc Surg 26:299–302

4. Lindholt JS, Juul S, Fasting H, et al (2005) Screening for abdominal aortic aneurysms: single centre randomised controlled trial. BMJ 330:750
5. Fleming C, Whitlock EP, Beil TL, et al (2005) Screening for abdominal aortic aneurysm: a best-evidence systemic review for the U.S. Preventive Services Task Force. Ann Intern Med 142:203–211
6. Golledge J, Powell JT (2007) Medical management of abdominal aortic aneurysm. Eur J Vasc Endovasc Surg 34:267–273
7. Poldermans D, Boersma E, Bax JJ, et al (1999) The effect of bisoprolol on perioperative mortality and myocardial infarction in high risk patients undergoing vascular surgery. N Engl J Med 341:1789–1794
8. Brady AR, Fowkes FG, Thompson SG, et al (2001) Aortic aneurysm diameter and risk of cardiovascular mortality. Arterioscler Thromb Vasc Biol 21:1203–1207
9. UK Small Aneurysms Trial Participants (2007) The long term prognosis of patients with small abdominal aortic aneurysms following surveillance: 12-year final follow-up of patients enrolled in the UK Small Aneurysm Trial. Br J Surg 94:702–708
10. Lederle FA, Johnson GR, Wilson SE, et al (2002) Rupture rate of large abdominal aortic aneurysms in patients refusing or unfit for elective repair. JAMA 287:2968–29732
11. UK Small Aneurysm Trial Participants (1998) Mortality results for randomised controlled trial of early elective surgery or ultrasonographic surveillance for small abdominal aortic aneurysms. Lancet 352:1649–1655
12. EVAR trial participants (2005) Endovascular Aneurysm Repair Versus Open Repair in Patients with Abdominal Aortic Aneurysm (EVAR Trial 1): Randomized Controlled Trial. Lancet 365:2179–86
13. Choke E, Cockerill G, Wilson WRW, et al (2005) A Review of Biological Factors Implicated in Abdominal Aortic Aneurysm Rupture. Euro J Vasc Endovasc Surg 30:227–244
14. Strachan DP (1991) Predictors of death from aortic aneurysms among middle-aged men: the Whitehall study. Br J Surg 78:701–704
15. Hackam DG, Thiruchelvam D, Redelmeier DA (2006) Angiotensin-converting enzyme inhibitors and aortic rupture: a population-based case-control study. Lancet 368:659–665
16. Wilson WRW, Evans J, Bell PRF (2005) HMG-CoA Reductase Inhibitors (Statins) Decrease MMP-3 and MMP-9 Concentrations in Abdominal Aortic Aneurysms. Euro J Vasc Endovasc Surg 30:259–262
17. Evans J, Powell JT, Schwalbe E, et al (2007) Simvastatin Attenuates the Activity of Matrix Metalloprotease-9 in Aneurysmal Aortic Tissue. Euro J Vasc Endovasc Surg 34:302–303
18. Kazi M, Thyberg J, Religa P (2003) Influence of intraluminal thrombus on structural and cellular composition of abdominal aortic aneurysm wall. J Vasc Surg 38:1283–1292
19. Dawson J, Vig S, Choke E, et al (2007) Medical optimisation can reduce morbidity and mortality associated with elective aortic aneurysm repair. Euro J Vasc Endovasc Surg 33:100–104
20. Veith FJ, Ohki T, Lipsitz EC, et al (2003) Endovascular grafts and other catheter-directed techniques in the management of ruptured abdominal aortic aneurysms. Semin Vasc Surg 16:326–331
21. Dutton RP, Mackensie CF, Scalea TM (2002) Hypotensive resuscitation during active haemorrhage: impact on in-hospital mortality. J Trauma 52:1141–1146
22. Brady AR, Gibbs JS, Greenhalgh RM, et al (2005) POBBLE trial investigators. Perioperative beta-blockade (POBBLE) for patients undergoing infrarenal vascular surgery: results of a randomized double-blind controlled trial. J Vasc Surg 41:602–609
23. Mangano DT, Leyug EL, Wallace A, et al (1996) Effect of atenolol on mortality and cardiovascular morbidity after noncardiac surgery. N Engl J Med 335:1713–1721
24. Schouten O, van Urk H, Feringa HH, et al (2005) Regarding "Perioperative beta-blockade (POBBLE) for patients undergoing infrarenal vascular surgery: results of a randomized double-blind controlled trial". J Vasc Surg 42:825
25. Kertai MD, Boersma E, Westerhout CM, et al (2004) Association between long-term statin use and mortality after successful abdominal aortic aneurysm surgery. Am J Med 116:96–103

26. Leurs LJ, Visser P, Laheij RJ, et al (2006) Statin use is associated with reduced all-cause mortality after endovascular abdominal aortic aneurysm repair. Vascular 14:1–8
27. Tilson MD, et al (1992) Aneurysms and atherosclerosis. Atherosclerosis 85(1):378–9
28. Thompson RW (1996) Basic science of abdominal aortic aneurysms: emerging therapeutic strategies for an unresolved clinical problem. Curr Opin Cardiol 11:504–518
29. Rijbroek A, Moll FL, Von Dijk HA, et al (1994) Inflammation in the abdominal aortic aneurysm wall. Eur J Vasc Surg 8:41–46
30. Brophy CM, Reilly JM, Smith GJ, et al (1991). The role of inflammation in nonspecific abdominal aortic aneurysm disease. Ann Vasc Surg 5:229–233
31. Freestone T, Turner RJ, Coady A, et al (1995) Inflammation and matrix metalloproteinases in the enlarging abdominal aortic aneurysm. Arterioscler Thromb Vasc Biol 15:1145–1151
32. Lopez-Candales A, Holmes DR, Liao S, et al (1997) Decreased vascular smooth muscle cell density in medial degeneration of human abdominal aortic aneurysms. Am J Pathol 150:993–1007
33. Anidjar S, Dobrin PB, Eichorst M, et al (1992) Correlation of inflammatory infiltrate with the enlargement of experimental aortic aneurysm. J Vasc Surg 16:139–147
34. Busuttil RW, Abou-Zamzam AM, Machleder HI, et al (1980) Collagenase activity of the human aorta: a comparison of patients with and without abdominal aortic aneurysms. Arch Surg 115:1373–1378
35. Dobrin PB, Mrkvicka R (1994) Failure of elastin or collagen as possible critical connective tissue alterations underlying aneurysmal dilatation. Cardiovasc Surg 2:484–488
36. Satta J, Haukipuro K, Kairaluoma MI, et al (1997) Aminoterminal propeptide of type III procollagen in the follow-up of patients with abdominal aortic aneurysms. J Vasc Surg 25:909–915
37. Newman KM, Malon AM, Shin RD (1994) Matrix metalloproteinases in abdominal aortic aneurysm: characterization, purification, and their possible sources. Connect Tissue Res 30:265–276
38. Szekaneez Z, Shah MR, Pearce WH, et al (1994) Human atherosclerotic abdominal aortic aneurysms produce (IL)-6 and interferon-gamma but not IL-2 and IL-4: the possible role for IL-6 and interferon-gamma in vascular inflammation. Agents and Actions 42:159–162
39. Juvonen J, Surcel HM, Satta J, et al (1997) Elevated Circulating Levels of Inflammatory Cytokines in Patients with Abdominal Aortic Aneurysm. Arterioscler Thromb Vasc Biol 17:2843–2847
40. Longo GM, Xiong W, Greiner TC, et al (2002) Matrix metalloproteinases 2 and 9 work in concert to produce aortic aneurysms. J Clin Invest 110:625–32
41. Pyo R, Lee JK, Shipley JM, et al (2000) Targeted gene disruption of matrix metalloproteinase-9 (gelatinase B) suppresses development of experimental abdominal aortic aneurysms. J Clin Invest 105:1641–9
42. Allaire E, Forough R, Clowes M, et al (1998) Local overexpression of TIMP1 prevents aortic aneurysm degeneration and rupture in a rat model. J Clin Invest 102:1413–20
43. Newman KM, Malon AM, Shin RD (1994) Matrix metalloproteinases in abdominal aortic aneurysms: characterization, purification, and their possible sources. Connect Tissue Res 30:265–276
44. Irizarry E, Newman KM, Gandhi RH, et al (1993) Demonstration of intestinal collagenase in abdominal aortic aneurysm disease. J Surg Res 54:571–574
45. Newman KM, Ogata Y, Malon AM, et al (1994) Identification of matrix metalloproteinases 3 (stromelysin-1) and 9 (gelatinase B) in abdominal aortic aneurysm. Arterioscler Thromb 4:1315–1320
46. Wilson WRW, Anderton M, Schwalbe EC, et al (2006) Matrix Metalloproteinase-8 and -9 Are Increased at the Site of Abdominal Aortic Aneurysm Rupture. Circulation 113:438–445
47. Allaire E, Forough R, Clowes M, et al (1998) Local over- expression of TIMP-1 prevents aortic aneurysm degeneration and rupture in a rat model. J Clin Invest 102:1413–1420
48. Choke E, Thompson MM, Dawson J, et al (2006) Abdominal Aortic Aneurysm Rupture Is Associated With Increased Medial Neovascularization and Overexpression of Proangiogenic Cytokines. Arterioscler Thromb Vasc Biol 26:2077–82

49. Cronenwett JL, Sargent SK, Wall MH, et al (1990) Variables that affect the expansion rate and outcome of small abdominal aortic aneurysms. J Vasc Surg 11:260–269
50. Thompson RW, Parks WC, et al (1996) Role of matrix metalloproteinases in abdominal aortic aneurysms. Ann N Y Acad Sci 800:157–174
51. Ong G, Thomas BJ, Mansfield AO, et al (1996) Detection and widespread distribution of Chlamydia pneumoniae in the vascular system and its possible implications. J Clin Pathol 49: 102–106
52. Meijer A, Roholl PJM, Gielis-Proper SK, et al (2000) Chlamydia pneumoniae in vitro and in vivo: a critical evaluation of in situ detection methods. J Clin Pathol 53:904–910
53. Cicconi V, Mannino S, Caminiti G, et al (2004) Salmonella Aortic Aneurysm: Suggestions for Diagnosis and Therapy Based on Personal Experience. Angiology 55:701–705
54. Gregory AK, Yin NX, Capella J, et al (1996) Features of autoimmunity in the abdominal aortic aneurysm. Arch Surg 131:85–88
55. Miller FJ Jr, Sharp WJ, Fang X, et al (2002) Oxidative stress in human abdominal aortic aneurysms: a potential mediator of aneurysm remodeling. Arterioscler Thromb Vasc Biol 22:560–565
56. Yajima N, Masuda M, Miyazaki, et al (2002) Oxidative stress is involved in the development of experimental abdominal aortic aneurysm: a study of transcription profile with complementary DNA microarray. J Vasc Surg 36:379–85
57. Verloes A, Sakalihasan N, Koulischer L, et al (1995) Aneurysms of the abdominal aorta: familial and genetic aspects in three hundred thirteen pedigrees. J Vasc Surg 21:646–655
58. Majumder PP, St Jean PL, Ferrell RE, et al (1991) On the inheritance of abdominal aortic aneurysm. Am J Hum Genet 48: 164–170
59. Shibamura H, Olson JM, van Vlijmen-Van Keulen C, et al (2004) Genome scan for familial abdominal aortic aneurysm using sex and family history as covariates suggests genetic heterogeneity and identifies linkage to chromosome 19q13. Circulation 109:2103–2108
60. Shanks N, Joplin KH (1999) Redundant Complexity: A Critical Analysis of Intelligent Design in Biochemistry. Philosophy of Science 66: 268–298
61. Boucek RJ, Gunja-smith Z, Noble NL, et al (1983) Modulation by Propranolol of the lysyl cross-links in aortic elastin and collagen of the aneurysm prone turkey. Biochem Pharmacol 32:275–80
62. Moursi MM, Beebe HG, Messina LM, et al (1995). Inhibition of Aortic Aneurysm development in blotchy mice by beta adrenergic blockade independent of altered lysyl oxidase activity. J Vasc Surg 21:792–800
63. Propranolol Aneurysm Trial Investigators (2002) Propranolol for small abdominal aortic aneurysms: results of a randomized trial. J Vasc Surg 35:72–9
64. Dobrin PB, Baumgartner N, Anidjar S, et al (1996) Inflammatory aspects of experimental aneurysms. Effect of methylprednisolone and cyclosporine. Ann N Y Acad Sci 800:74–88
65. Ricci MA, Strindberg G, Slaiby JM, et al (1996) Anti-CD-18 monoclonal antibody slows experimental aortic aneurysm expansion. J Vasc Surg 32:301–7
66. Holmes DR, Petrinec D, Wester W, et al (1996) Indometacin prevents elastase induced abdominal aortic aneurysms in the rat. J Surg Res 63:305–9
67. Franklin IJ, Walton LJ, Greenhalgh RM, et al (1999) The influence of Indometacin on the metabolism and cytokine secretion of human aneurysmal aorta. Euro J Vasc Endovasc Surg 18:35–42
68. Powell JT, Greenhalgh RM, Ruckley CV, et al (1996) The UK Small Aneurysm Trial. Ann N Y Acad Sci 800:249–251
69. Boyle JR, McDermott E, Crowther M, et al (1998) Doxycycline inhibits elastin degradation and reduced metalloproteinase activity in a model of aneurysmal disease. J Vasc Surg. 27:354–61
70. Vammen S, Lindholt JS, Andersen PL, et al (2001) Antibodies against Chlamydia pneumoniae predict the need for elective surgical intervention on small abdominal aortic aneurysms. Euro J Vasc Endovasc Surg 22:165–8

71. Lindholt JS, Vammen S, Lind I, et al (1999) The progression of lower limb atherosclerosis is associated with IgA antibodies against Chlamydia pneumoniae. Euro J Vasc Endovasc Surg 18:527–9
72. Morrison M, Juvonen J, Biancari F, et al (2001) Use of doxycycline to decrease the rate of growth of abdominal aortic aneurysms: a randomized, double-blind, placebo-controlled pilot study. J Vasc Surg 34:606–610
73. Vammen S, Lindholt JS, Ostergaard L, et al (2001) Randomised double-blind placebo controlled trial of Roxithromycin for prevention of abdominal aortic aneurysm expansion. Br J Surg. 88:1066–1072
74. Baxter BT, Pearce WH, Waltke EA, et al (2002) Prolonged administration of Doxycycline in patients with small asymptomatic abdominal aortic aneurysms: report of a prospective (phase II) multicentre study. J Vasc Surg 36:1–12
75. Fisher JF, Mobasheri S (2006) Recent advances in MMP inhibitor design. Cancer Metastasis Rev 25:115–136
76. Nagashima H, Aoka Y, Sakomura Y, et al (2002) A 3-hydroxy-3-methylglutyryl coenzyme-A reductase inhibitor, cerivastatin, suppresses production of matrix metalloproteinase-9 in human abdominal aortic aneurysm wall. J Vasc Surg. 36:158–163
77. Kothe H, Dalhoff K, Rupp J (2000) Hydroxymethylglutyryl coenzyme-A reductase inhibitors modify the inflammatory response of human macrophages and endothelial cells infected with Chlamydia Pneumoniae. Circulation 101:1760–3
78. Schouten O, van Laanen JH, Boersma E, et al (2007) Statins are associated with a reduced infra-renal abdominal aortic aneurysm growth. Euro J Vasc Endovasc Surg 94:8–9

Regression of Abdominal Aortic Aneurysms through Pharmacologic Therapy

Koichi Yoshimura, Hiroki Aoki, Yasuhiro Ikeda, Akira Furutani, Kimikazu Hamano, and Masunori Matsuzaki

Summary Abdominal aortic aneurysm (AAA) is a common disease that eventually results in aortic rupture with high mortality. Although a pharmacologic therapy for AAA is eagerly awaited, the destruction of the aortic walls in AAA has been considered an irreversible process. Recently, we identified c-Jun N-terminal kinase (JNK) as a key molecule in the pathogenesis of AAA. JNK was highly activated in the aortic walls of AAA patients. In in vitro studies, JNK not only enhanced expression of matrix metalloproteinases (MMPs), but also reduced expression of biosynthetic enzymes for extracellular matrix (ECM). An AAA model induced by $CaCl_2$ in mice was accompanied by activation of JNK and MMP-9. Treatment with a specific JNK inhibitor, SP600125, completely prevented AAA formation. SP600125 also caused a significant reduction in aneurysmal diameter in established AAA. Surprisingly, SP600125 was effective in normalizing tissue architecture. Furthermore, treatment with SP600125 caused significant regression of angiotensin II-induced AAA in ApoE-null mice after its establishment. These data indicated that pharmacologic inhibition of JNK caused healing of aneurysmal tissue and regression of established AAA, providing a novel therapeutic option for treatment of AAA.

Keywords abdominal aortic aneurysm (AAA) · regression · pharmacologic therapy · c-Jun N-terminal kinase (JNK) · extracellular matrix (ECM)

K. Yoshimura (✉), H. Aoki, Y. Ikeda, and M. Matsuzaki
Department of Molecular Cardiovascular Biology, Yamaguchi University School of Medicine, 1-1-1 Minami Kogushi, Ube, Yamaguchi 755-8505, Japan
e-mail: yoshimko@yamaguchi-u.ac.jp

A. Furutani and K. Hamano
Department of Surgery and Clinical Science, Yamaguchi University Graduate School of Medicine, 1-1-1 Minami Kogushi, Ube, Yamaguchi 755-8505, Japan

M. Matsuzaki
Department of Medicine and Clinical Science, Yamaguchi University Graduate School of Medicine, 1-1-1 Minami Kogushi, Ube, Yamaguchi 755-8505, Japan

Introduction

Abdominal aortic aneurysm (AAA) is a common disease that is characterized by chronic inflammation and degradation of extracellular matrix (ECM) by proteolytic enzymes, such as matrix metalloproteinases (MMPs), and eventually progresses to aneurysmal rupture with a high mortality [1]. Because most of patients with AAA have no symptoms until the catastrophic events of the rupture, main purpose of treatment for patients with AAA is to prevent the aneurysmal rupture, thereby improving their prognosis. Current therapeutic options to prevent the rupture of AAA are limited to open aneurysm repair or endovascular repair. When these surgical treatments are not applicable, AAA is growing with increasing its diameter as well as rupture risk. It is widely accepted that AAA diameter is a major predictor of rupture. Therefore, a therapy that causes regression of AAA size would reduce the risk of rupture, provided that the disrupted tissue architecture is normalized. However, the destruction of aortic wall structure and the enlargement of aneurysm diameter have been considered irreversible processes. While an effective reduction in AAA size by non-surgical therapy has not been achieved, it was reported that a successful endovascular aneurysm repair caused the regression of human AAA [2]. This result strongly suggests that human AAA walls have the potential to regress when exacerbating factors are eliminated and/or tissue repair is reinforced.

We hypothesized that endovascular exclusion may block the effect of hemodynamic stress or humoral factors onto the vascular cells of AAA, thereby stopping destruction of extracellular matrix, and that regression of AAA may be achieved by inhibition of a critical signaling pathway in the pathogenesis of AAA. Actually, it was reported that plasma level of MMP-9 was significantly decreased after successful endovascular repair [3]. Based on this hypothesis, we have conducted a series of experiments to demonstrate the regression of established AAAs in mice through a pharmacologic inhibition of c-Jun N-terminal kinase (JNK) [4]. Here, we summarize our recent findings regarding the regression of AAA through pharmacologic therapy.

Activation of JNK in Human AAA Walls

First, we screened for activation of several signaling pathways in human AAA. We observed a significant increase in JNK phosphorylation in human AAA walls compared with the level in the non-aneurysmal aorta (Fig. 1a). Recent studies indicate that JNK is involved in a number of cellular stress responses and also in the signaling of inflammation [5]. Other mitogen-activated protein kinases, such as ERK or p38, did not show such an obvious activation in AAA. Consistent with previous reports [1], protein expression level of MMP-9 was significantly increased in AAA (Fig. 1a). Interestingly, active JNK levels showed a highly positive correlation with levels of MMP-9 expression in human AAA walls. Histological analysis

Fig. 1 Role of JNK on pathogenesis of AAA. (**a**) Protein expression of phosphorylated JNK and MMP-9 in human control aorta and AAA, determined by western blotting and gelatin zymography, respectively. (**b**) Effect of SP600125 (SP), a specific JNK inhibitor, on secretion of MMP-9 from human AAA ex vivo culture, determined by gelatin zymography. (**c**) Role of JNK on mRNA expression of LOX in vascular smooth muscle cells. JNK was either activated by over-expression of constitutively active MKK7 and JNK1, or inhibited by a peptide inhibitor (JNK-I). Data are means ± SE (n=6) as shown by fold change compared with GFP or control. **P<0.01, compared with GFP or control. §§P<0.01, compared with a control peptide (TAT). (Modified from [4])

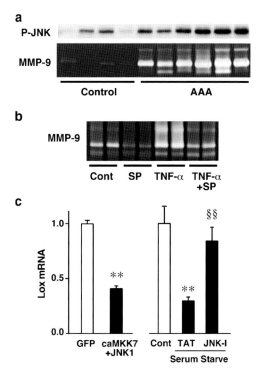

demonstrated the colocalization of JNK activity and MMP-9 in human AAA walls. Most of active JNK was localized in macrophages, which are known to secrete proinflammatory cytokines and MMP-9, and some active JNK was localized in vascular smooth muscle cells, which synthesize ECM and secrete MMP-2. These results prompted us to further investigate the link between JNK activation and ECM degradation in AAA.

Role of JNK in ECM Metabolism

To obtain further insight into the role of JNK in AAA, we screened for JNK-dependent genes in VSMCs. We performed the DNA microarray analysis, following the specific activation of JNK by active MKK7 or specific inhibition of JNK by dominant negative JNK in VSMCs. According to our analysis, JNK upregulates the positive regulators of MMP-9, including inducible nitric oxide synthase, interleukin-1alpha, lipocalin-2 and MMP-9 itself. Using *ex vivo* culture of human AAA walls, we found that SP600125 [6], a specific JNK inhibitor, significantly suppressed the secretion of MMP-9. Tumor necrosis factor (TNF)-α, a proinflammatory cytokine, caused a large increase in MMP-9 secretion from human AAA tissues, which was also abrogated by a JNK inhibitor (Fig. 1b). It is widely accepted that MMPs, particularly MMP-9, cause the loss of critical ECM components, including collagen and elastin, thereby leading to AAA development [7,8]. Pharmacologic inhibition of MMPs has been shown to reduce the expansion rate of AAA in animal models [9,10] and in early clinical trials [11,12].

On the other hand, we have found that JNK downregulates the critical enzymes for ECM biosynthesis, such as lysyl hydroxylase (PLOD), prolyl 4-hydroxylase (P4H) and lysyl oxidase (LOX). Consistent with our array data, we found that inhibition of JNK restored the expression of both P4H and LOX, which was reduced by JNK activation (Fig. 1c). As we and others reported, the local activity of LOX, which is essential for stabilization of collagen and elastin fibers [13], was decreased during the development of AAA [4,10]. These findings suggested that impairment in ECM biosynthesis and stabilization is involved in the progression of AAA and that JNK may enhance AAA formation not only by enhancing degradation of ECM but also by attenuating connective tissue repair.

Prevention of AAA Development by JNK Inhibition

To test our hypothesis using *in vivo* model, we created AAA in mice by periaortic application of 0.5 M $CaCl_2$ [14]. Following the application of $CaCl_2$, mice were treated with SP600125 or vehicle for 10 weeks. We chose pharmacologic inhibition of JNK, because of the practical relevance of a pharmacologic approach in humans with AAA. Treatment of mice with SP600125 completely abrogated the increase in aortic diameter induced by $CaCl_2$ and significantly reduced both phospho-c-Jun, a marker of JNK activity, and MMP-9 level. Histological examination revealed that SP600125 prevented the destruction of aortic tissue architecture and also reduced inflammatory cell infiltration into the aneurysmal tissue, suggesting that JNK inhibition abrogates proinflammatory cascades in AAA. These findings demonstrate that pharmacologic inhibition of JNK is an effective therapeutic option to prevent the development of AAA.

Regression of AAA by JNK Inhibition

Our *in vitro* data suggested that inhibition of JNK not only suppresses a degradation pathway, but also restores a biosynthetic pathway of ECM. Therefore, we examined whether pharmacologic inhibition of JNK can cause regression of already established AAA, which presumably requires tissue repair including active ECM biosynthesis. Periaortic application of $CaCl_2$ caused significant dilation of the aorta after 6 weeks. We started SP600125 or vehicle treatment at 6 weeks after $CaCl_2$

treatment and continued for an additional 6 weeks. Vehicle treatment resulted in no significant changes in aneurysmal diameters, indicating that the CaCl$_2$-induced AAA was fully established at the 6 weeks and maintained for an additional 6 weeks. Surprisingly, inhibition of JNK by SP600125 caused a striking reduction in aneurysmal diameters (Fig. 2a). On histological analysis, disruption and flattening of elastic lamellae were observed in the aneurysmal wall 6 weeks after CaCl$_2$ treatment. Vehicle treatment for an additional 6 weeks resulted in no significant changes. However, SP600125 restored a wavy morphology with less disruption of elastic lamellae, indicating that JNK inhibition enhances the repair of tissue architecture (Fig. 2b).

Furthermore, we tested the effect of JNK inhibitor in another AAA model created by continuous infusion of angiotensin II in apolipoprotein E-null mice [15]. This model is advantageous because AAA develops in the suprarenal aorta, allowing us to monitor the aneurysmal diameter by ultrasonography. Our serial ultrasonographic studies demonstrated that SP600125 caused a striking reduction of AAA induced by angiotensin II in ApoE-null mice. These data demonstrated for the first time that pharmacologic treatment with the JNK inhibitor causes regression of established AAA in animal models.

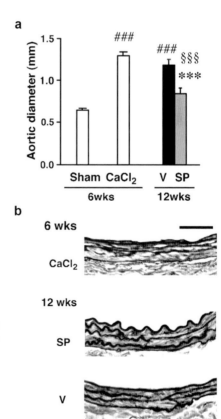

Fig. 2 Regression of AAA by JNK inhibition. (a) Effect of JNK inhibitor on the size of AAA. Aortic diameters were determined 6 weeks after the CaCl$_2$ treatment or sham operation, and after an additional 6 weeks of vehicle (V) or SP600125 (SP) treatment. Data are means ± SE (n=9). ***P<0.001, compared with those at 6 weeks after the CaCl$_2$ treatment. §§§P<0.001, compared with vehicle treatment. ###P<0.001, compared with sham operation. (b) Effect of JNK inhibitor on the tissue architecture. Morphology of elastic lamella is shown by elastica van Gieson staining. Bars indicate 40 μm. (Modified from [4])

Fig. 3 Central role of JNK in the balance between tissue repair and degradation. (**a**) JNK activates the tissue degradation and simultaneously suppresses the ECM biosynthesis and the tissue repair, resulting in the development and progression of AAA. (**b**) Inhibition of JNK ameliorates abnormal metabolism of ECM and enhances tissue repair, resulting in regression and healing of AAA

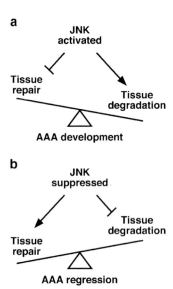

Conclusion

We have identified JNK as a critical factor causing abnormal ECM metabolism by enhancing tissue degradation and by inhibiting tissue repair in AAA (Fig. 3a). We found that specific inhibition of JNK not only suppresses the destruction, but also restores the ECM biosynthesis and tissue repair, resulting in the regression of AAA in two mouse models (Fig. 3b). Thus, pharmacologic inhibition of JNK may provide a novel therapeutic option for treatment of human AAA [4,16–18]. We hope that a JNK-inhibition strategy would help to improve the prognosis of AAA patients by expanding the non-surgical therapeutic options.

Acknowledgments The authors gratefully thank all the people who helped in this project. This work was supported in part by Grants-in-aid for Scientific Research (KAKENHI) from the Japan Society for the Promotion of Science (KY, HA, and MM) and a grant from the Sankyo Company to the Department of Molecular Cardiovascular Biology, Yamaguchi University School of Medicine.

References

1. Thompson RW, Geraghty PJ, Lee JK (2002) Abdominal aortic aneurysms: basic mechanisms and clinical implications. Curr Probl Surg 39:110–230
2. Buth J, Harris P (2005) Endovascular Treatment of Aortic Aneurysms ed. Rutherford R B Elsevier, Philadelphia, 1452–1475
3. Sangiorgi G, D'Averio R, Mauriello A, et al (2001) Plasma levels of metalloproteinases-3 and -9 as markers of successful abdominal aortic aneurysm exclusion after endovascular graft treatment. Circulation 104:I288–295

4. Yoshimura K, Aoki H, Ikeda Y, et al (2005) Regression of abdominal aortic aneurysm by inhibition of c-Jun N-terminal kinase. Nat Med 11:1330–1338
5. Manning AM, Davis RJ (2003) Targeting JNK for therapeutic benefit: from junk to gold? Nat Rev Drug Discov 2:554–565
6. Bennett BL, Sasaki DT, Murray BW, et al (2001) SP600125, an anthrapyrazolone inhibitor of Jun N-terminal kinase. Proc Natl Acad Sci USA 98:13681–13686
7. Pyo R, Lee JK, Shipley JM, et al (2000) Targeted gene disruption of matrix metalloproteinase-9 (gelatinase B) suppresses development of experimental abdominal aortic aneurysms. J Clin Invest 105:1641–1649
8. Baxter BT (2004) Could medical intervention work for aortic aneurysms? Am J Surg 188:628–632
9. Petrinec D, Liao S, Holmes DR, et al (1996) Doxycycline inhibition of aneurysmal degeneration in an elastase-induced rat model of abdominal aortic aneurysm: preservation of aortic elastin associated with suppressed production of 92 kD gelatinase. J Vasc Surg 23:336–346
10. Huffman MD, Curci JA, Moore G, et al (2000) Functional importance of connective tissue repair during the development of experimental abdominal aortic aneurysms. Surgery 128:429–438
11. Mosorin M, Juvonen J, Biancari F, et al (2001) Use of doxycycline to decrease the growth rate of abdominal aortic aneurysms: a randomized, double-blind, placebo-controlled pilot study. J Vasc Surg 34: 606–610
12. Baxter BT, Pearce WH, Waltke EA, et al (2002) Prolonged administration of doxycycline in patients with small asymptomatic abdominal aortic aneurysms: report of a prospective (Phase II) multicenter study. J Vasc Surg 36:1–12
13. Kagan HM, Li W (2003) Lysyl oxidase: properties, specificity, and biological roles inside and outside of the cell. J Cell Biochem 88:660–672
14. Longo GM, Xiong W, Greiner TC, et al (2002) Matrix metalloproteinases 2 and 9 work in concert to produce aortic aneurysms. J Clin Invest 110:625–632
15. Daugherty A, Manning MW, Cassis LA (2000) Angiotensin II promotes atherosclerotic lesions and aneurysms in apolipoprotein E-deficient mice. J Clin Invest 105:1605–1612
16. Thompson RW (2005) Aneurysm treatments expand. Nat Med 11:1279–1281
17. Yoshimura K, Aoki H, Ikeda Y, et al (2006) Identification of c-Jun N-terminal kinase as a therapeutic target for abdominal aortic aneurysm. Ann N Y Acad Sci 1085:403–406
18. Aoki H, Yoshimura K, Matsuzaki M (2007) Turning back the clock: regression of abdominal aortic aneurysms via pharmacotherapy. J Mol Med 85:1077–1088

Gene Therapy for Treating Abdominal Aortic Aneurysm using Chimeric Decoy Oligodeoxynucleotides Against NFκB and ets in a Rabbit Model

Takashi Miyake

As current therapy to treat abdominal aortic aneurysm (AAA), and particularly to manage small AAA, is limited to elective surgical repair, we explored less invasive molecular therapy by simultaneous inhibition of the transcription factors, NFκB and ets, using a decoy strategy.

Initially, we examined the expression of NFκB and ets in human AAA sample. Of importance, both transcription factors were markedly activated in the neck of AAA. In addition, immunohistochemical staining also demonstrated an increase in NFκB- and ets-positive cells in outer aneurysm wall.

Thus, we focused on the simultaneous inhibition of both NFκB and ets and employed chimeric decoy oligodeoxynucleotides (ODN) containing consensus sequences of both transcription factors binding sites. Inhibitory effects of chimeric decoy ODN on matrix metalloproteinases (MMP)-1 and MMP-9 expression was confirmed by ex vivo experiments using the organ cultured human aorta.

To examine the regressive effect of chimeric decoy ODN in a rabbit already-formed AAA model, transfection by wrapping a delivery sheet containing decoy ODN around the aneurysm was performed one week after incubation with elastase. Treatment with chimeric decoy ODN significantly regressed the size of AAA in a dose-dependent manner. Preservation of elastic fibers was observed with chimeric decoy ODN treatment, accompanied by a reduction of MMP-2 and MMP-9 and induction of macrophage apoptosis, leading to inhibition of macrophage accumulation. Regression of AAA was also associated with an increase in elastin and collagen type I and III synthesis in the aneurysm wall.

Minimally invasive molecular therapy targeted to the inhibition of NFκB and ets is expected to be useful for AAA through the re-balance of matrix synthesis and degradation.

T. Miyake (✉)
Department of Clinical Gene Therapy, Graduate School of Medicine,
Osaka University, Osaka, Japan.

Simulation Study of Aortic Valve Function Using the Fluid-structure Interaction Finite Element Method

Seiryo Sugiura, Susumu Katayama, Nobuyuki Umetani, and Toshiaki Hisada

Summary The aortic root, with its characteristic morphology, has attracted the interest of researchers in both clinical and basic sciences, and the emergence of aortic root replacement surgery has further increased the significance of such studies. In addition to clinical observations, both experimental and theoretical studies have attempted to elucidate the dynamics of the aortic root; however, to date, most of these studies have dealt with simplified models of the aortic root, and are thus not readily applicable to clinical settings. Recently, 3-D finite element analyses of the aortic root have been reported, in which realistic shapes of both aorta and valve leaflet were modeled. So far, however, only a few studies have taken into consideration the effect of blood flow, an essential component of aortic root dynamics, due the difficulty in computation. We have developed a computational program for fluid-structure interaction analysis based on the arbitrary Lagrangian-Eulerian finite element method, and applied it to the simulation of aortic root dynamics. The results suggest the importance of vortex formation in the sinus of Valsalva in the smooth closure of the aortic valve.

Keywords finite element method · fluid-structure interaction analysis · aortic root · sinus of Valsalva

Introduction

Although the molecular bases have been clarified in some specific diseases, hemodynamic and mechanical stimuli are still recognized as the major initiators or modulators in the genesis and development of aortic root diseases, and thus,

---

S. Sugiura (✉), S. Katayama, N. Umetani, and T. Hisada
Department of Human and Engineered Environmental Studies, Graduate School of Frontier Sciences, The University of Tokyo, Kashiwanoha 5-1-5, Kashiwa-shi, Chiba 277-8563
e-mail: Sugiura@k.u-tokyo.ac.jp

are the targets of prevention strategies and treatments. Because the hemodynamics of the aortic root is heavily influenced by its shape as well as the pumping function of the heart, researchers have focused their attention on the functional impact of the characteristic morphology of the aortic root. In particular, interest on the shape of the sinus of Valsalva can be traced back to work by Leonardo da Vinci in the 16th century [1]. More recently, a series of model studies have promoted our understanding in this field [2–4]. Bellhouse and Talbot observed that the closing of the valve started during the deceleration phase of the aortic flow in the presence of a sinus cavity, and that the absence of sinuses increased the retrograde flow [3].

To explain such observations, theoretical considerations have been proposed. To investigate the dynamics of valve opening and the motion of the leaflet during the early phase of ejection, numerical analyses were carried out in a two-dimensional model [5,6]. Similarly, to investigate valve closing, van Steenhoven et al. used a mathematical model of the 2-D aortic root to show that deceleration of flow causes a motive force for valve closure, and verified this with an in vitro experiment [4]. Although these studies have helped us to understand the principle of the operation of the aortic valve, it may be hard to apply the knowledge obtained from such simplified models to clinical settings where detailed information on the 3D distributions of flow, stresses and/or strains are eagerly needed to understand the disease process and design optimal surgical treatments.

3D simulations of aortic root dynamics based on the finite element method have attempted to meet such requirements, but in most of the studies, including those on the abdominal aorta, the deformation of the wall in response to the increment in pressure was calculated and, so far, only a few studies have analyzed the fluid structure interaction, which, in fact, is the essential component of aortic root dynamics [7,8].

We have developed a robust finite element method in which fluid and structure are strongly coupled, and applied it to the multi-physics simulation of the heart [9–12]. In this paper, after reviewing preceding modeling work, we will introduce our strategy for finite element modeling of the aortic root dynamics based on fluid-structure interaction analysis.

Previous Studies

Experimental and Clinical Observations

In late 1960's, Bellhouse developed an experimental setup in which the motion of cusps made of nylon net impregnated with silicone rubber could be seen in a rigid aorta made from Perspex. They compared the two sets of Perspex tubes with or without sinuses, and found that, without sinuses, the cusps remained in the upright position (aligned with the wall) until the late phase of ejection and did not close until the reversal flow reached 23% of the forward flow, while valves with sinuses closed with only 4% regurgitation. Based on the simultaneous measurement of flow velocity in the sinuses, they found that the vortices in the sinuses persists after the main stream starts to decelerate and produce a thrust on the cusps to close them [2].

van Steenhoven et al. [4] carried out a similar study in a two dimensional flow channel. They also found that the reduction of the size of the sinus delayed the closure of the valves, but they rather questioned the role of vortex formation in the sinus as the motive force of valve closure and proposed that a simplified quasi-one-dimensional description of the flow, combined with an assumption of constant pressure on the sinus side of the cusp, can give a good qualitative approximation of the cusp motion in the initial phase of valve closure. They also reported that, in the case of high Strouhal number (St = $R/(U\tau)$, where R sinus radius, U peak systolic velocity, and τ deceleration time), the cusps underwent bending deformation, and were thus subject to a high stress but the entire cusp rotated around its point of attachment in the physiological case with low St. More recently, Fries et al. [13] studied the valve motion of porcine aortic valves that had been operated on with the David I (without sinus) and Yacoub (with neo-sinus) techniques in the test circuit. They found that the cusps in the tube graft (David I) remained wide open until the late phase of ejection and closed very rapidly, thus confirming the earlier observation. A similar study was performed by Erasmi et al. [14] who reported that the reimplantation technique (without a sinus) caused the largest deformation in the cusp compared with the remodeling technique or the native aortic root.

Similar observations were made in clinical settings. In a study comparing the opening and closing characteristics of the aortic valve after a valve sparing procedure, it was shown that the valve in the tube graft remained fully open until the late phase of ejection (characterized by the small slow closing displacement (SCD)) and then closed with high closing velocity [15]. A large SCD in the tube graft group was also reported by Leyh et al. [16], but the closing velocity was smaller with the tube graft used in this study. The reason for this discrepancy is not clear, but other hemodynamic factors such as the function of the heart may also affect the opening and the closure of the aortic valve.

Recent advancement in magnetic resonance imaging technology has made it possible to non-invasively map the aortic flow velocity, thus providing mechanistic information on the function of aortic valves. Using such technology, Markl et al. compared the flow pattern between healthy volunteers and patients after David reimplantation with a cylindrical graft and two versions of neo-sinus recreation [17]. Interestingly, although the creation of neo-sinus enhanced the vortex formation, normal vorticity was found without the sinuses. They postulated that the vortex formation is not predominantly determined by the mechanical and morphological properties of the sinus, but more related to the aortic flow dynamics.

Taken together, both experimental and clinical studies with their own advantages have provided important information; however, we still do not have a comprehensive view of aortic root dynamics.

Finite Element Analysis for the Study of Aortic Root Dynamics

3-D finite element modeling can be used not only for the verification of basic assumption by comparison with the clinical data, but also for the optimal design of the graft. For the latter purpose, Grande-Allen computed the stress in the leaflet for various morphologies of the aortic root, and concluded that the creation of a pseudo-sinus can greatly reduce the abnormal stress in the cylindrical graft [18]. However, because this simulation was done by applying only the pressure, and thus ignoring the effect of blood flow, we could not gain an insight into the dynamics of aortic valve closure. The same group reported the fluid-structure interaction analysis of blood flow and the motion of the valve leaflet in a 3-D finite element model of the aortic root, but some unphysiological assumptions were introduced to complete the computation [7]. On the other hand, using the fictitious-domain method, de Hart et al. [8] demonstrated the essential role of the vortex in sinuses for the smooth operation of the aortic valve, but, again, their computation was carried out with an unphysiologically low Reynolds number (900) due to the numerical instabilities inherent in the algorithm.

Our group has developed a strongly coupled fluid-structure interaction finite element analysis program [19] based on the arbitrary Lagrangian-Eulerian (ALE) method, and applied it to the multi-physics heart simulator [9–12]. This program enables us to compute the valve motion with the blood flow, the Reynolds number of which is as high as that in the human aorta (~3500).

In the following section, we will introduce our approach to the simulation analysis of aortic root dynamics based on this method.

ALE Finite Element Method for the Analysis of Aortic Root Dynamics

Finite Element Model and Boundary Conditions

As a first attempt to analyze aortic root dynamics, we modeled the proximal portion of the ascending aorta with a rigid straight tube. The fluid (blood) domain was modeled by tetrahedral finite elements with four velocity nodes and four pressure nodes. For the structural part (valve leaflets), we used Discrete Kirchhoff Triangular (DKT) shell elements with anisotropic material properties to reflect the fiber orientation [20].

Because only the short segment of the aorta was modeled, the rest of the systemic circulation was represented by a three-element Windkessel model of circulation. To the proximal end, we applied the prescribed time-varying pressure wave form simulating physiological left ventricular pressure (LVP) (Fig. 1).

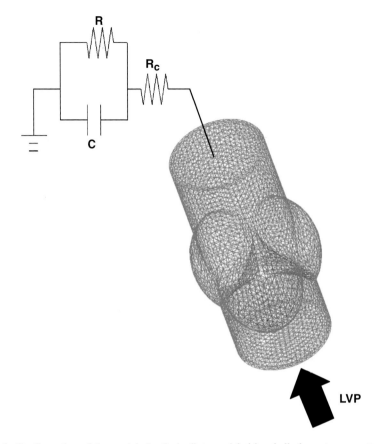

Fig. 1 Configuration of the model. Aortic leaflets modeled by shell elements were attached to the short segment of aorta with sinuses of Valsalva. A three-element Windkessel model of the systemic circulation was connected to the distal end and the time-varying pressure wave form simulating physiological left ventricular pressure was applied to the proximal end

Formulation

The Navier-Stokes equation was described and discretized in ALE coordinates with Streamline-Upwind/Petrov-Galerkin (SUPG), Pressure-Stabilizing/Petrov-Galerkin (PSPG), and Least-Squares Incompressibility Constraint (LSIC) stabilization terms. The structural governing equation in the total Lagrangian form was discretized. Then, the fluid and structural matrix equations were assembled while the nodes on the interface were shared by the fluid and structural elements, so that the velocities of both domains were identical at the common nodes. The assembled matrix equation is simultaneously solved without distinction of fluid and solid. This approach is classified as the so-called strong coupling method [19].

In the heart valve problem, movement of the fluid-structure interface introduces an excessive ALE mesh distortion and the resultant degradation of element performance. To circumvent this problem, our group has developed an automatic mesh reconnecting algorithm, which enhanced the power of our fluid-structure interaction analysis code without the high additional costs of re-meshing.

Preliminary Results

In response to the change in pressure applied to the proximal side, the aortic valves opened and closed smoothly with small regurgitant flow (2%). Notably, the vortex formation started at early phase of ejection coinciding with the initiation of the valve closure (Fig. 2A). Furthermore, the blood flow in the sinus formed a clockwise vortex, and thus seemed to push valves and facilitate closure.

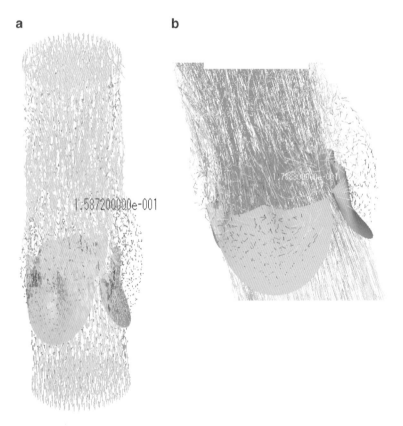

Fig. 2 Simulation results. (**a**) blood flow in the aorta and the motion of leaflets during the early phase of ejection. (**b**) Close-up view showing vortex formation in the sinus

Discussion

We have applied a strongly coupled fluid-structure interaction finite element analysis program [19] based on the arbitrary Lagrangian-Eulerian (ALE) method to the study of aortic root dynamics, and successfully reproduced vortex formation in the sinus of Valsalva. Although vortex formation seemed to facilitate the smooth closure of the aortic valves, a comparison of the dynamics between models with and without sinuses is definitely required to obtain conclusive evidence. The elastic behavior of the aortic wall should also be taken into consideration. Furthermore, we are planning to combine the aortic model to our multi-physics heart simulator [9–12] to simulate a more realistic condition. With such improvements, clinically applicable simulation of aortic root dynamics can be realized.

Acknowledgement This study was supported by a grant for Core Research for Evolutional Science and Technology from Japan Science and Technology Bureau (JST).

References

1. Robicsek F (1991) Leonardo da Vinci and the sinuses of valsalva. Ann Thorac Surg 52:328–335
2. Bellhouse BJ, Bellhouse FH. (1968) Mechanism of closure of the aortic valve. Nature 217:86–87
3. Bellhouse BJ, Talbot L (1969) The fluid mechanics of the aortic valve. J Fluid Mech 35:721–735
4. van Steenhoven AA, van Dongen MEH. (1979) Model studies of the closing behaviour of the aortic valve. J Fluid Mech 90:21–32
5. Swanson WM, Clark RE (1973) Numerical-graphical determination aortic valve leaflet motion during systole. Circ Res 32:42–48
6. Hung TK, Schuessler GB (1977) An analysis of the hemodynamics of the opening of aortic valves J Biomech 10:597–606
7. Nicosia MA, Cochran RP, Einstein DR, et al (2003) A coupled fluid-structure finite element model of the aortic valve root. J Heart Valve Dis 12:781–789
8. De Hart J, Peters GWM, chreurs PJGS, et al (2003) A three-dimensional computational analysis of fluid–structure interaction in the aortic valve. J Biomech 36:103–112
9. Watanabe H, Hisada T, Sugiura S, et al (2002) Computer Simulation of Blood Flow, Left Ventricular Wall Motion and Their Interrelationship by Fluid-Structure Interaction Finite Element Method. JSME Internatl J Series C 45:1003–1012
10. Watanabe H, Sugano T, Sugiura S, et al (2004) Finite element analysis of ventricular wall motion and intra-ventricular blood flow in heart with myocardial infarction. JSME Internatl J Series C 47:1019–1026
11. Watanabe H, Sugiura S, Hisada T (2003) Finite element analysis on the relationship between left ventricular pump function and fiber structure within the wall. JSME Internatl J Series C 46:1330–1339
12. Watanabe H, Sugiura S, Kafuku H, et al (2004) Multi-physics simulation of left ventricular filling dynamics using fluid-structure interaction finite element method. Biophys J 87:2074–2085
13. Fries R, Graeter T, Aicher D, et al (2006) In vitro comparison of aortic valve movement after valve-preserving aortic replacement. J Thorac Cardiovas Surg 132:32–37

14. Erasmi A, Sievers H-H, Scharfschwerdt M, et al (2005) In vitro hydrodynamics, cusp-bending deformation, and root distensibility for different types of aortic valve-sparing operations: Remodeling, sinus prosthesis, and reimplantation. J Thorac Cardiovas Surg 130:1044–1049
15. De Paulis R, De Matteis GM, Nardi P, et al (2001) Opening and closing characteristics of the aortic valve after valve-sparing procedure using a new aortic root conduit. Ann Thorac Surg 72:487–494
16. Leyh RG, Schimidke C, Sievers H-H, et al (1999) Opening and closing characteristics of the aortic valve after different types of valve-preserving surgery. Circulation 100:2153–2160
17. Markl M, Draney MT, Miller DC, et al (2005) Time-resolved three-dimensional magnetic resonance velocity mapping of aortic flow in healthy volunteers and patients after valve-sparing aortic root replacement. J Thorac Cardiovas Surg 130:456–463
18. Grande-Allen KJ, Cochran RP, Reinhall PG, et al (2000) Re-creatrion of sinuses is important for sparing the aortic valve: a finite element study. J Thorac Cardiovas Surg 119:753–763
19. Zhang Q, Hisada T (2001) Analysis of Fluid-Structure Interaction Problems with Structural Buckling and Large Domain Changes by ALE finite element method. Comput Methods Appl Mech Engrg 190:6341–6357
20. Swanson WM, Clark RE (1974) Dimensions and geometric relationship of the human aortic valve as a function of pressure. Circ Res 35:871–882

Symposium 1
State of Arts: Stent Graft for Thoracic Aorta

Long Term Results of Aortic Arch Repair Using Stent Grafting Technique

Masaaki Kato, Kazuo Shimamura, Toru Kuratani,
Hiroshi Takano, and Nobukazu Ohkubo

Abstract

Objective: This report elucidates the long-term safety and effectiveness of aortic arch repair using stent graft from our 12 years experience.

Methods: Open stent grafting technique: From 1994 to 2004, 126 patients (mean age 67.8 years) with different aortic arch pathologies (57 dissections and 69 aneurysms) were operated with open stent grafting technique. Under deep hypothermic circulatory arrest with selective cerebral perfusion, the stent graft was delivered through the transected proximal aortic arch and arch replacement was performed with 4 branched prosthesis.

TPEG (Transluminally Placed Endovascular Grafting) with bypass to neck vessels: From 1997 to 2007, 26 patients (mean age 65.3 years) with different distal arch pathologies (17 dissections and 9 aneurysms) were operated with TPEG with bypass to neck vessels. 6 aorto-carotid and/or subclavian bypass, 4 axillary-carotid and/or axillary bypass, and 16 carotid-subclavian bypass were performed prior to TPEG.

Results: Open stent grafting technique: Operative mortality was 3.2%. Perioperative morbidity included 7 (5.6%) strokes, 3 (2.4%) paraplegias, 5 (3.9%) transient parapalesis. Sixty three percent of the patients were extubated within 24 hours. In long term follow up (mean 60.4 ± 36.5 months, maximum 153 months), survival was 81.1%, 63.3% and 53.7% at 1, 5 and 8 years. Five (3.9%) late endoleaks were observed but treated with successful additional endovascular repair. Freedom from endoleaks was 98.0%, 91.1%, 91.1% for 1, 5 and 8year respectively.

TPEG with neck bypass: Operative mortality was 3.8%. Perioperative morbidity included 1 (3.8%) minor stroke, 1 (3.8%) pulmonary embolism and 3 (11.5%) endoleak (type I). In follow up, no endoleak was observed.

M. Kato and N. Ohkubo
Department of Cardiovascular Surgery, Morinomiya Hospital, Osaka, Japan

K. Shimamura, T. Kuratani, and H. Takano
Department of Cardiovascular Surgery, Osaka General Medical Center, Osaka, Japan

Conclusion: Long term observation showed safety and good durability of hybrid procedures using stent graft for aortic arch disease. These technique could be an attractive treatment option for aortic arch aneurysm with distal extension and aortic dissection requiring aortic arch repair.

Endovascular Repair of Thoracic Aortic Aneurysms

Katsuhiko Oka

Abstract Endovascular repair of thoracic aortic diseases is one of the hopeful alternatives to conventional open surgery that is sometimes responsible for the tragic complications. Conventional total arch repair of aortic aneurysm is requiring cardiopulmonary bypass and deep hypothermic circulatory arrest. Despite recent improvements in surgical technique, total arch repair still has significant morbidity and mortality.

But endovascular repair is not requiring CPB and DHCA. Therefore, the morbidity and mortality in stent-grafting is lower than surgical arch repair.

We have applied endovascular repair for 92 cases of thoracic aortic diseases since Dec 2001. At first in our team, stent-grafts with fenestration were located from ascending aorta (zone 0) for the arch aneurysm. We would introduce the present endovascular stent-grafting in detail.

K. Oka (✉)
Kyoto Prefectural University of Medicine, Japan

Current Endograft Therapy of Type B Aortic Dissection

Sidney L. Kahn and Michael D. Dake

Summary Over the last decade, the emergence of endovascular therapies provides an alternative to both open surgery and medical therapy in the management of patients with type B aortic dissection. The benefits of this new approach are perhaps most apparent in the reported experience with endografts used in the setting of acute dissection complicated by rupture, organ malperfusion, rapidly expanding false lumen, or unremitting pain. Successful placement of an aortic endograft across the entry tear(s) of the dissection with obliteration of this communication(s) to the false lumen and re-direction of blood flow via the true lumen exclusively is an increasingly valuable treatment strategy in selected patients with complicated dissection. The results in this setting compare very favorably with those reported for traditional open surgical therapy with less morbidity and risk of paraplegia. Currently, global consensus does not yet support the extension of endograft use to include patients with uncomplicated acute dissection or chronic dissection.

Keywords Aorta · Dissection · Endograft · Therapy · Entry Tear

Background of Aortic Dissection

Despite a dramatic reduction in the mortality attributable to cardiovascular disease in the United States over the last five years, it remains the leading cause of mortality in Western society and is on the rise in developing nations.[1] Aortic dissection surpasses AAA rupture 2 to 3 fold as the most common aortic injury with an incidence of 2.6 to 3.5 per 100,000 person years.[2,3,4,5] The male to female ratio of aortic

---

S.L. Kahn and M.D. Dake
University of Virginia Health System, Department of Radiology

M.D. Dake (✉)
University of Virginia Health System, Department of Radiology,
1215 Lee Street, Rm 1076, Charlottesville, VA 22908
e-mail: mdd2n@virginia.edu

dissection ranges from 2:1 to 5:1[2,6,7,8,9] with an average age of 63 as reported by the International Registry of Acute Aortic Dissection (IRAD).[31]

Aortic dissection results from disruption of the aortic intima and partial thickness of the media with entrance of blood into a longitudinal plane within the medial layer. While this is a property shared by all dissections, the subsequent course and extent are highly variable among patients. The proximal or distal (more common) propagation, involvement of aortic branches, resultant aneurysmal dilatation of the aorta, and the number of sites of communication between the true and false lumens varies from patient to patient.

Equally variable are the clinical sequelae of aortic dissection with potentially grave consequence. Expansion of the false lumen may lead to aneurysmal dilatation and rupture, itself the most common cause of death related to aortic dissection.[23] Moreover, expansion of the false lumen may compress the true lumen, thereby compromising flow to its dependent branch vessels. Experimental work by Chung et al. suggests the ratio of inflow and outflow in the true and false lumens is responsible for these sequelae.[10,11]

The heterogeneous nature of aortic dissection undoubtedly lends itself to the complex medical, surgical, and endovascular approaches to treatment.

Stanford Type B Aortic Dissections

Classification and Natural History

The Stanford system classifies dissections as type A involving the ascending aorta (DeBakey types II and III) or type B (DeBakey type III) consisting of any dissection that does not involve the ascending aorta. Among these, type B dissections account for between 30–40% of all dissections.[12,31] In the absence of treatment, survival rates for patients with type B dissections are 91% at 1 month, 89% at 1 year, and 80% at 5 years.[43] Between 20 and 28% of type B dissections ultimately develop thoracic aortic aneurysms requiring repair in a follow up period of 40–50 months. Fatal rupture of the aorta occurs in up to 18% of patients.[13,14,15]

Traditionally, type B dissections have been characterized as either acute or chronic with chronic dissections being those that are greater than 2 weeks of age. It is estimated that approximately one third of dissections are chronic at the time of diagnosis.[2,16] However, this classification has fallen out of favor more recently, as it provides little information in determining which patients would benefit from surgical or endovascular therapy as opposed to traditional medical therapy. More recently, type B dissections have been more appropriately characterized as "complicated" or "uncomplicated" based on expansion/imminent rupture, development of pseudoaneurysm of the false lumen, persistent thoracic pain, drug resistant hypertension, the development of malperfusion syndrome, and the anatomical considerations of the dissection.[32,17,46,23] It is estimated that approximately 20% of cases are complicated at the time of diagnosis, requiring either endovascular or surgical repair.[42,31,18] Commonly, type B dissections are stratified as acute onset complicated, acute onset uncomplicated, and chronic, although many chronic dissections are technically uncomplicated.

Anatomy and Risk Factors

Type B dissections most commonly originate just distal to the ligamentum arteriosum, presumably because of the greater hemodynamic stress at this location.[2,19] Among the various risk factors for type B dissection, systemic hypertension remains at the forefront, occurring in up to 70% of all dissections.[2,31,8,20] This stands in contrast to type A dissections, which tend to occur in a younger cohort, are less associated with hypertension (36%[2,21,8,20]), and are more frequently associated with underlying congenital conditions (e.g., Marfan's, Ehlers-Danlos) that predispose the vasculature to medial necrosis.

Traditional Approach to Uncomplicated Type B Dissections

Surgical Therapy

Conventional teaching has advocated the use of medical therapy with a tailored antihypertensive regimen as the initial approach to uncomplicated type B dissections.[21] Surgery has traditionally been reserved for complicated dissections, despite high associated morbidity and mortality. While it shares the high technical success rate of endovascular repair, surgical options remain encumbered by substantial post-operative morbidity and mortality. Earlier reports of operative mortality range from 6–67%[46,22] to 35–50%[23,24] after open surgical repair. While more recent reports have estimated this risk at 4.8–8.8%, this remains unacceptable.[45,25,26,27] The wide variation in these estimates is partially attributable to the discrepancy in risk between acute and chronic cases, with substantially higher associated operative risk in the acute setting. Respiratory failure, renal failure, and spinal ischemia are common morbidities. It is reported that a 14 to 67% risk of irreversible spinal cord injury or post-operative mortality is associated with surgical management.[32,28,29,30]

Medical Therapy

Medical therapy, as a first line approach to uncomplicated type B aortic dissections, is based on the fact that provided alone, it confers a relatively good short-term prognosis with 85% of patients surviving their initial hospital stays.[31] The reported 30-day mortality of uncomplicated type B dissection is 10% versus 30% in complicated cases involving extremity ischemia, renal failure, visceral ischemia, or contained rupture.[31] Unfortunately, the long-term outcomes offered by medical therapy alone are suboptimal with a reported 50% mortality at 5 years and delayed expansion of the false lumen in 25% patients at 4 years.[32] This expansion of the false lumen predisposes patients to aortic rupture or retrograde migration of the dissection plane with involvement of the ascending aorta and a consequent increased mortality rate.[32] Aneurysmal dilatation of the aorta is observed in more than 20% of patients managed medically at follow up.[42] Although calculated from retrospective data, Kaplan-Meier curves derived for 80 patients at the Hamburg and Rostock University Hospitals yield a 12 month mortality of 27.5% with conventional therapy alone versus a 5.1% in a similar set of patients treated with endovascular stent-grafts.[32]

Paradigm Shift: Endovascular Repair of Type B Aortic Dissection

General

Landmark studies by Dake et al. and Nienaber et al. in 1999 demonstrated endovascular stent-grafting as an effective alternative for the management of acute type B dissections.[28,29] However, as recently as 2005, the consensus remained that uncomplicated type B dissections are best managed medically as surgical and endovascular interventions offered no validated benefit over medical regimens in stable patients.[33] In Circulation 2005, Tsai et al. acknowledge the potential for endovascular treatment of uncomplicated type B dissections in the future, but state that "patients with uncomplicated aortic dissections confined to the descending aorta are at present best treated with medical therapy."[34]

Despite such consensus, the propagation of non-invasive imaging modalities and the improved life expectancy of patients with aortic dissection have shifted the focus to long-term outcomes. The efficacy of endovascular therapy, reduced procedure time, low intraoperative complications, and relatively lower associated morbidity have won favor with investigators in recent years as a potential first line treatment for uncomplicated type B aortic dissections. Moreover, the prospect of aortic remodeling after dissection and the prevention of future aneurysm formation and rupture has reinvigorated this debate.

Successful endovascular therapy with stent-graft therapy is predicated on adequate coverage and sealing of the entry site.[32] Experimental models indicate that proper placement of the stent-graft results in thrombosis of the false lumen, an event known to be associated with an improved prognosis, whereas patency of the false lumen is associated with late mortality.[2,35,36,37] A properly positioned stent-graft with occlusion of the proximal tear will result in decompression of the false lumen and re-expansion of the true lumen. Thrombosis of the false lumen typically occurs within 3 months.[28] Aortic remodeling occurs quickly after stent-graft placement [2,28] and has the potential to reverse branch vessel ischemia and inhibit re-canalization of the thrombosed false lumen.[2]

Timing of Intervention

The optimal time for endovascular intervention of all type B dissections is a contentious topic. A retrospective study performed by Bortone et al. in 2002[46] strongly defends immediate intervention, as defined as procedures performed within 2 weeks of the initial diagnosis. Stent-graft placement was successful in all patients referred for intervention within the first two weeks. Conversely, 8 of 13 (61.5%) patients referred after two weeks' time failed to undergo stent graft placement because of a tortuous course of the dissection and multiple sites of communication between the true and false lumens. Moreover, a thick and fibrotic dissection flap may impede adequate stent-graft expansion.[2] Despite these impediments, successful stent-graft management in chronic dissections treated after 2 weeks has been reported by multiple groups.[2,45,32,38,39]

As described previously, rapid intervention in the acute phase is also associated with its own complications as the adventitia and dissection flap are weak and vulnerable to injury induced by placement of a stent-graft. Various groups have argued for greater than 1 week to 1 month elapsed time prior to intervention.[42,43] Interestingly, the inclusion criteria of the INSTEAD trial (discussed below) require intervention between 2 and 52 weeks thereby rendering the possibility that this study may shed light on the subject. While it is probable that the optimal time for intervention lies in the subacute phase, the exact timing should give deference to the patient's underlying morbidities and the specific anatomical considerations of the dissection.

Recent Work

While there is a paucity of investigative literature directly assessing the role of endovascular stent-grafting as a means for intervention in uncomplicated type B aortic dissections, multiple studies have included patients in this cohort, thereby providing insight to this prospect.

Hausegger et al. (2001)[40]

In this study, 5 patients with type B aortic dissection were treated successfully with endovascular stent-grafting. However, of these 5, only 2 met the criteria to be considered uncomplicated cases treated only for aneurysmal dilatation to prevent future rupture. One patient had a dissection with no identifiable re-entry site. In both patients, stent-grafting resulted in thrombosis of the false lumen. In the patient with no distal re-entry site, a 5 mm inconsequential dissection that remained stable for 36 months (last follow-up) developed just distal to the prosthesis. Both patients experienced transient hypertension that was controlled within 48–72 hours. Otherwise, no immediate or late complications developed in these patients. Furthermore, there was no subsequent aneurysm development in the uncomplicated patients, although development of a 4 cm aneurysm was reported in one of the complicated patients, who initially had presented with intractable pain and stenosis of the right renal artery. Although limited by a small sample size, use of a single device (Talent™), and a single institution, this study does support the prophylactic use of endovascular stent grafts in uncomplicated type B dissections.

Palma et al. (2002)[41]

Between 1996 and 2001, a total of 198 patients with aortic disease were enrolled in the study, with 70 patients treated for dissection. Of these 70, 58 had type B dissections, but only 3 of the 58 patients were performed electively for uncomplicated cases (large flow volume in the false lumen). Although the analysis in this study did not independently assess uncomplicated cases, it did demonstrate the efficacy of stent-graft placement for type B dissection and a low complication rate. Technical success as defined by exclusion of the false lumen was 92.9%. Complications included conversion to open surgery (2), procedural-related deaths (2), delayed left subclavian artery compromise (1), stroke (2), access site vessel injury (2), DVT (1), mild transient renal failure (15), wound/dialysis catheter infection (3), and fever (15). No paraplegia occurred despite the use of multiple stent-grafts in many patients. The authors conclude that endovascular stent grafting is an ideal option for both complicated and uncomplicated type B dissections with considerably less risk than conventional open surgery.

Kato et al. (2002)[42]

This study enrolled 38 patients between 1997 and 2002. There were 28 type B dissections, 8 of which were acute uncomplicated, 6 were acute complicated, and 14 were chronic type B dissections. Although 8 were classified as uncomplicated, inclusion criteria mandated that these patients have one of three criteria: i) descending thoracic aorta > 40 mm at onset, ii) descending thoracic aorta >50 mm at any time, or iii) observation of growth of an ulcer-like projection. 24 patients underwent treatment within 1 month of diagnosis, while 14 underwent treatment between 1 month and 30 years after the initial diagnosis.

While the primary purpose of this study was to investigate the longer term outcomes of stent-graft therapy for dissection, several important observations regarding uncomplicated dissections were made. The immediate outcome mortality (≤ 30 days), intraoperative complications (stroke, intimal injury), and postoperative complications (aorta and non-aorta related) were significantly higher in patients with complicated dissection compared to those with uncomplicated dissection. Although there were no late mortalities in this study, late complications (aorta and non-aorta related) were comparable between complicated and uncomplicated patients. Interestingly, there were no early or late mortalities in patients treated with chronic dissections and the early and late complication rates were significantly lower in chronic cases as compared to acute cases (complicated or uncomplicated). The authors contend that uncomplicated cases are best treated after one month as the adventitia and aortic flap are very fragile and thus subject to complications in the acute phase. The results of this study support the use of stent-grafting for prevention of potentially fatal complications in appropriately selected patients.

Totaro et al. (2002)[43]

In a study conducted at single institution in Italy between 2000 and 2001, 32 patients with either descending thoracic aneurysm or type B dissection underwent endovascular stent-graft repair. 25 patients with type B dissection were enrolled, 5 underwent repair in the acute phase (defined as <2 weeks) and 20 underwent repair during the subacute phase (defined as > 2weeks and < 2 months). All patients had chronic hypertension and none presented with an underlying congenital condition.

Although limited by use of a single stent-graft (Excluder™), the study yielded a 100% technical success rate and a low complication rate, including 1 intraoperative retrograde dissection, 10 cases of primary endoleak (7 successfully treated, 3 with subsequent spontaneous thrombosis), 4 cases of fever, and 8 cases of access site infection. As demonstrated in numerous other studies, there were no cases of paraplegia. To reduce complications, the authors argue strongly for a week of antihypertensive therapy prior to intervention in the setting of acute, uncomplicated type B aortic dissection. Unlike most, this group utilizes endovascular therapy as a first-line approach for all uncomplicated type B dissections.[44]

Shimono et al. (2002)[45]

Between 1997 and 2000, 37 patients with acute and chronic aortic dissection were enrolled in a retrospective, single institution trial in Japan. The goals set forth by the investigators for treating acute onset dissections were to lower the complication risk of an emergent operation and to prevent subsequent aneurysmal dilatation of the aorta necessitating future intervention in the chronic phase. Of the 37 patients,

24 were acute onset and 13 were chronic. Within the acute subset, 8 were without complication. As with Kato et al., the decision to treat an acute uncomplicated case was based on aortic size >40 mm, as this is deemed to be at high risk for aneurysmal dilatation in the chronic phase. Chronic dissections were treated if they contained ulcer like projections or maintained a maximal diameter greater than 50 mm. Complicated cases received intervention on the day of admission, but uncomplicated cases were treated electively following extensive evaluation with non-invasive imaging.

Follow-up evaluation with CT was performed at 4 weeks, 3 and 6 months, then yearly thereafter, with a mean follow-up time of 24.5 months. There was a single death, likely related to pre-operative morbidities. No early complications were observed in the uncomplicated acute onset group in contrast to 18.8% in the complicated acute-onset group and 7.7% in the chronic dissection group. Endoleaks were more common in the acute onset cases than the chronic cases, despite a high rate of false lumen thrombosis at the initial post-operative CT. The primary success rate as defined by thrombosis of the false lumen and absence of an endoleak was highest in the chronic dissection group (100%) as compared to the complicated acute onset (93.3%) and uncomplicated acute onset (87.5%) patients. As noted in the early follow-up, complications related to the stent-graft were more common in the complicated acute onset group (20%) relative to the uncomplicated acute onset group (12.5%) and the chronic dissection group (0%). Additionally, final CT imaging (mean follow-up 21.5 months) revealed complete or partial thrombosis of the false lumen in 94.4% overall with a reduction (≥5 mm) in aortic diameter observed in 87.5% of uncomplicated acute onset patient in contrast to 93.3% of acute onset complicated patients and 84.6% of chronic dissections.

As demonstrated in other studies, this work further validates the efficacy of stent-grafting not only in the chronic phase, but also in acute uncomplicated dissection cases.

Bortone et al. (2002)[46]

Although primarily designed to assess the impact of delayed vs. immediate intervention for type B dissection and post-traumatic aortic pseudoaneurysms, a study by Bortone et al. in 2002 included data on stent-graft placement for 7 acute and 5 chronic type B dissections performed electively. While not explicitly stated, the elective nature of these procedures suggests that these were not complicated dissections as described above. A single mortality was reported on a patient with substantial co-morbidities that received delayed stent-graft intervention. A reported 100% technical success rate was obtained on the patients who underwent endovascular repair within 2 weeks of the initial diagnosis. As reported in other trials, a low complication rate was attained with no immediate life threatening complications and three major complications (1 acute renal failure and 2 lower limb ischemia). There were no cases of paraplegia. Closure of the false lumen was attained in all patients at 3 months. The high technical success and clinical efficacy and relatively low complication rate in this study provided the foundation for the later INSTEAD trial (discussed below).

The INSTEAD Trial (2006)[32]

The European INSTEAD trial is a 7 center, prospective randomized trial investigating the use of stent-grafts with adjunctive medical therapy versus medical therapy alone in patients with uncomplicated type B aortic dissections. Although limited by the exclusive use of the Medtronic Talent™ stent-graft, this trial is the most comprehensive study to date evaluating the use of stent-grafts in this population. 136 patients will be enrolled in the study and followed at 3, 12, and 24 month intervals. Patients must have an uncomplicated type B dissection with a patent false lumen older than 14 days and less than 52 weeks since dissections less than 2 weeks of age often thrombose spontaneously thus conferring a better prognosis, while those greater than 52 weeks of age are less amenable to intervention secondary to a thickened, fibrotic dissection flap.[2,32]

Preliminary data presented by Dr. Christoph Nienaber at the Charing Cross 28th International Symposium in April of 2006 demonstrated a near 100% success rate with respect to closure of the tear entry (1 patient failure) and no intraprocedural mortality. True lumen enlargement occurred in 92% and reduction of the false lumen in 63% of patients. Although 16% of patients in the stent-graft arm experienced overall aortic expansion of greater than 5 mm, none required surgical or endovascular revision prior to discharge. At 3 months there were 5 deaths in the stent-graft arm, but only two attributable to dissection or other aortic complications, and 0 deaths in the medical therapy group. At 3 months, 52% of patients had total thrombosis of the false lumen, while 27% had partial thrombosis.

It is likely that a greater difference between the stent-graft and medical therapy patient subsets will become evident when data is analyzed from the 12 and 24 month intervals. The trial is due for publication in 2006 and will likely bear substantial influence on the use of stent-grafts in uncomplicated type B dissections.

Discussion

The initial work of Dake et al.[28] in 1999 illustrating the efficacy of endovascular stent-grafting for acute aortic dissection challenges the traditional medical and surgical approaches to this devastating disease, bringing less invasive therapy to the forefront of the physician's arsenal. In conjunction, Nienaber et al.'s comparison of surgical and stent-graft outcomes highlighted the shortcomings of surgery for chronic dissections, revealing a statistically significant higher rate of operative morbidity and mortality.[29] Combined, these studies laid the foundation for numerous subsequent studies evaluating the merits of stent-grafts for acute and chronic dissections.

Despite this trend, the use of medical therapy as a first-line treatment in uncomplicated type B dissections has remained relatively unchallenged. This in no small part reflects the adequacy of this tactic for short-term results. However, the fact that approximately 20–28% of patients with uncomplicated dissections are ultimately complicated by aneurysmal dilatation underscores the need for a long-term focus.[13,14,15]

The studies reviewed in this article demonstrate that endovascular stent-grafting is a promising approach to uncomplicated type B dissections, reducing short-term mortality and avoiding late complications, including re-dissection, rupture, and late surgical repair.[39]

Essential to successful stent-grafting is proper patient selection, appropriate technique, and optimal timing. Preliminary work, suggests that patients with uncomplicated dissections should be stratified based on their likelihood of long term complications. Shimono et al. and Kato et al.'s attempt at risk stratification based on aortic diameter supports this practice.[45,39] Moreover appropriate case selection based on the anatomical considerations of the dissection (tortuosity, involvement of branch vessels, etc.), the presence of adequate peripheral access, and the assessment of patient co-morbidities is essential for optimizing successful results.

Appropriate technique mandates proximal occlusion of the entry tear for decompression of the false lumen. Moreover, minimization of the angle between the inferior portion of the stent-graft and the native aortic wall minimizes iatrogenic stress thus lowering subsequent aneurysmal dilatation.[42] It is without doubt that innovations in stent-graft technology with greater customization and flexibility will improve technical outcomes.

Finally, while a general consensus has not been reached, preliminary work suggests that the timing of intervention plays a role in the success of endovascular repair, with optimal intervention conducted at some point in the subacute phase.

The promising results of endovascular repair indicate that in conjunction with medical therapy, its role as a first-line therapeutic and prophylactic approach to uncomplicated aortic dissection will strengthen in the near future. The exact role of endovascular therapy in this setting will be elucidated as the results from the INSTEAD trial and future randomized trials come to fruition. It is conceivable that as this new role is validated, conventional surgery's role will be relegated to those cases subsequently complicated by failure of thrombosis of the false lumen and persistent communication between the true and false lumens.

References

1. Nienaber CA, Eagle MA (2003) Aortic Dissection: New Frontiers in Diagnosis and Management. Circulation 108:628–635
2. Wang DS, Dake MD (2006) *Abrams' Angiography Interventional Radiology*. Second Edition. pp 415–455

3. Bickerstaff LK, Pairolero PC, Hollier LH, et al (1982) Thoracic aortic aneurysms: a population based study. Surgery 92:1103–1108
4. Clouse WD, Hallett JW Jr, Schaff HV, et al (2004) Acute aortic dissection: population-based incidence compared with degenerative aortic rupture. Mayo Clin Proc 79:176–180
5. Meszaros I, Morocz J, Szlavi J, et al (2000) Epidemiology and clinicopathology of aortic dissection. Chest 117:1271–1278
6. Coady MA, Rizzo JA, Goldstein LJ, et al (1999) Natural history, pathogenesis, and etiology of thoracic aortic aneurysms and dissections. Cardiol Clin 17:615–635; vii
7. DeBakey ME, McCollum CH, Crawford ES, et al (1982) Dissection and dissecting aneurysms of the aorta: twenty-year follow-up of five hundred twenty-seven patients treated surgically. Surgery 92:1118–1134
8. Hirst AE Jr, Johns VJ Jr, Kime SW Jr (1958) Dissecting aneurysm of the aorta: a review of 505 cases. Medicine (Baltimore) 37:217–279
9. Wilson SK, Hutchins GM (1982) Aortic dissecting aneurysms: causative factors in 204 subjects. Arch Pathol Lab Med 106:175–180
10. Chung JW, Elkins C, Sakai T, et al (2000) True-lumen collapse in aortic dissection. I. Evaluation of causative factors in phantoms with pulsatile flow. Radiology 21:87–98
11. Chung JW, Elkins C, Sakai T, et al (2000) True-lumen collapse in aortic dissection. II. Evaluation of treatment methods in phantoms with pulsatile flow. Radiology 214:99–106
12. Sorensen HR, Olsen H (1964) Ruptured and dissecting aneurysms of the aorta. Incidence and prospects of surgery. Acta Chir Scand 128:644–650
13. Grabenwoger M, Fleck T, Czerny M, et al (2003) Endovascular stent graft placement in patients with acute thoracic aortic syndromes. European Journal of Cardio-thoracic Surgery 23:788–793
14. Juvonen T, Ergin MA, Galla JD, et al (1999) Risk factors for rupture of chronic type B dissections. J Thorac Cardiovasc Surg 17:776–86
15. Genoni M, Paul M, Jenn R, et al (2001) Chronic Beta blocker therapy improves outcome and reduces treatment costs in chronic type B dissection. Eur J Cardiothorac Surg 19:606–610
16. Spittell PC, Spittell JA Jr, Joyce JW, et al (1993) Clinical features and differential diagnosis of aortic dissection: experience with 236 cases (1980 through 1990). Mayo Clin Proc 68:642–651
17. Nienaber CA, Ince H, Weber F, et al (2003) Emergency stent-graft placement in thoracic aortic dissection and evolving rupture. J Card Surg 18:464–70
18. Schor JS, Yerlioglu ME, Galla JD, et al (1996) Selective management of acute type B aortic dissection: long-term follow-up. Ann Thorac Surg 61:1339–41
19. Wheat MW Jr (1987) Acute dissection of the aorta. Cardiovasc Clin 17:241–262
20. Larson EW, Edwards WD (1984) Risk factors for aortic dissection: a necroscopy study of 161 cases. Am J Cardiol 53:849–855
21. Wheat MW Jr (1980) Current status of medical therapy of acute dissecting aneurysms of the aorta. World J Surg 4:563–9
22. Svensson LG (1997) Natural history of aneurysms of the descending thoracoabdominal aorta. J Card Surg 12:279–284
23. Miller DC (1992) Acute dissection of the descending thoracic aorta. Chest Surg Clin North Am 2:347–55
24. Elefteriades JA, Hartleroad J, Gusberg RJ, et al (1992) Long-term experience with descending aortic dissection: The complication-specific approach. Ann Thorac Surg 53:11–21
25. Estrera AL, Rubenstein FS, Miller CC, et al (2001) Descending thoracic aortic aneurysm: surgical approach and treatment using the adjuncts cerebrospinal fluid and distal aortic perfusion. Ann Thorac Surg 72:481–486
26. Kouchoukos NT, Masetti P, Rokkas CK, et al (2001) Safety and efficacy of hypothermic cardiopulmonary bypass and circulatory arrest for operations on the descending thoracic and thoracoabdominal aorta. Ann Thorac Surg 72:699–708
27. Coselli JS, LeMaire SA, Miller CC, et al (2000) Mortality and paraplegia after thoracoabdominal aneurysm repair: a risk factor analysis. Ann Thorac Surg 69:409–414

28. Dake MD, Kato N, Mitchell RS, et al (1999) Endovascular stent-graft placement for the treatment of acute aortic dissection. NEJM 340:1546–52
29. Nienaber CA, Fattori R, Lung G, et al (1999) Nonsurgical reconstruction of thoracic aortic dissection by stent-graft placement. NEJM 340:1539–45
30. Fattori R, Caldarera I, Rapezzi C, et al (2000) Primary endoleakage in endovascular treatment of the thoracic aorta: importance of intraoperative transesophageal echocardiography. J Thorac Cardiovasc Surg 120:490–5
31. Hagan PG, Nienaber CA, Isselbacher EM, et al (2000) The international registry of aortic dissection (IRAD): new insights into an old disease. JAMA 283:897–903
32. Nienaber CA, Zannetti S, Barbieri B, et al (2005) INvestigation of STEnt grafts in patients with type B Aortic Dissection: Design of the INSTEAD trial—a prospective, multicenter European randomized trial. Am Heart J 149:592–9
33. Mukherjee D, Eagle KA (2005) Aortic Dissection—An Update. Curr Probl Cardiol 30:287–325
34. Tsai TT, Nienaber CA, Eagle KA (2005) Acute Aortic Syndromes. Circulation 112;3802–3813
35. Erbel R, Oelert H, Meyer J, et al (1993) Effect of medical and surgical therapy on aortic dissection evaluated by transesophageal echocardiography. Implications for prognosis and therapy. The European Cooperative Study Group on Echocardiography. Circulation 87:1604–1615
36. Ergin MA, Phillips RA, Galla JD, et al (1994) Significance of distal false lumen after type A dissection repair. Ann Thorac Surg 57:820–824; discussion 825
37. Williams DM, Andrews JC, Marx MV, et al (1993) Creation of reentry tears in aortic dissection by means of percutaneous balloon fenestration: gross anatomic and histologic considerations. J Vasc Interv Radiol 4:75–83
38. Nienaber CA, Ince H, Petzsch M, et al (2003) Endovascular treatment of acute aortic syndrome. Supplement to Endovascular Today 12–15
39. Kato N, Hirano T, Shimono T, et al (2000) Treatment of chronic type B aortic dissection with endovascular stent graft placement. Cardiovasc Intervent Radiol 23:60–62
40. Hausegger KA, Tiesenhausen K, Schedlbauer P, et al (2001) Treatment of Acute Aortic Type B Dissection with Stent-Grafts. Cardiovasc Intervent Radiol 24:306–312
41. Palma JH, Marcondes de Souza JA, Rodrigues Alves CM, et al (2002) Self-Expandable Aortic Stent-Grafts For Treatment of Descending Aortic Dissections. Ann Thorac Surg 73:1138–42
42. Kato N, Shimono T, Hirano T, et al (2002) Midterm results of stent-graft repair of acute and chronic aortic dissection with descending tear: The complication-specific approach. J Thorac Cardiovasc Surg 124:306–12
43. Totaro M, Mazzesi G, Marullo AG, et al (2002) Endoluminal stent grafting of the descending thoracic aorta. Ital Heart J 3:366–369
44. Totaro M, Miraldi F, Fanelli F, et al (2001) Emergency surgery for retrograde extension of type B dissection after endovascular stent graft repair. Case report. European Journal of Cardio-thoracic Surgery 20:1057–1058
45. Shimono T, Kato N, Yasuda F, et al (2002) Transluminal Stent-Graft Placements for the Treatments of Acute Onset and Chronic Aortic Dissection. Circulation 106:I-241–I-247
46. Bortone AS, Schena S, D'Agostino D, et al (2002) Immediate Versus Delayed Endovascular Treatment of Post-Traumatic Aortic Pseudoaneurysms and Type B Dissections: Retrospective Analysis and Premises to the Upcoming European Trial. Circulation 106:234–240

Endovascular Treatment of Chronic Type B Aortic Dissection

Rossella Fattori

The optimal management of descending aortic dissection is controversial. Even though medical therapy demonstrated some early survival benefit with respect to surgical repair, no significant difference in long term outcome has been demonstrated.

Mortality is related either to retrograde progression of dissection with involvement of the proximal aorta or to expansion of the false lumen and formation of a thoracic aneurysm. Several reports in the literature analysed long-term outcome in patients with type B dissection, comparing medical with surgical therapy without evidence of a significant difference between the two groups. Five-year survival rates between 32%–72% have been reported because medical therapy alone cannot prevent the evolutive course of the disease. Recently, the development of endovascular therapy offers additional opportunity in the treatment of type B dissection as potential alternative to medical therapy and open surgical repair. The rationale of endovascular treatment of aortic dissection was originally based on evidence in the literature of protective effect of false lumen thrombosis against false lumen expansion and on the clinical observation that patients in the rare instance of spontaneous thrombosis of the false lumen have a better long-term prognosis than without it. Conversely, persistent perfusion of the false lumen has been identified as an independent predictor of progressive aortic enlargement and adverse long-term outcome. Closure of the entry tear of a type B dissection may promote both depressurisation and shrinkage of the false lumen, with subsequent thrombosis, fibrous transformation, remodelling and stabilization of the aorta. Published data confirm the technical feasibility and a relative low rate of complications with respect to surgical repair. However long-term follow-up and outcome information, in order to document the sustained benefit of endovascular repair, are still limited. With growing experience in endovascular stent-graft treatment, the spectrum of acute and midterm complications has broadened to include potentially disastrous events. Late aneurismal degeneration of the thrombosed false lumen has been reported, and also several case reports have highlighted the risk of retrograde extension of

---

R. Fattori (✉)
Cardiovascular Department – Radiology Unit – University Hospital S. Orsola, Bologna

the dissection into the ascending aorta, potentially caused by stent-graft induced intimal injury. Even though extension of dissection is known event in the course of type B dissection disease, wire or sheath manipulation during the endovascular procedure could increase the risk of this dreadful complication. Continuous progress in stent-graft technology, improving morphology and flexibility, may lead to more suitable stent-graft configuration for aortic dissection. However, these unexpected complications underline the particular fragility of the aortic wall and the need of careful selection criteria and rigorous follow-up. Before the responses of controlled randomized trials it will be difficult to provide certainties on which is the best timing and treatment modality with respect to acute and chronic forms.

Long-term Evolution of Type B Dissection and Endovascular Therapy Indications

Arturo Evangelista, Rio Aguilar, Teresa González-Alujas, Patricia Mahia, and José Rodríguez-Palomares

Summary The long-term evolution of type B aortic dissection has relatively high mortality or need for surgery, which approach 50% in 5 years. Some clinical predictive such as age, chronic obstructive pulmonary disease, hypertension and Marfan Syndrome factors have been associated with a high risk of complications. However, information obtained by imaging techniques has significant prognostic value. In addition to maximum aorta diameter, the combination of large entry tear size and true lumen compression or partial false lumen thrombosis is the best predictor of mortality and aortic dilatation. In these cases endovascular therapy should be considered in subacute phase. Treatment efficacy is greater in this phase than in chronic phase when the aorta is severely dilated and the intima is less elastic. Indications for stent grafting or surgery in the chronic phase are based on the size and growth of the dissecting aneurysm. Careful blood pressure control and annual follow-up by imaging techniques are necessary to prevent the aortic rupture, and elective endovascular therapy should be considered if aortic diameter exceeds 60 mm or increases significantly (> 5 mm/y).

General consensus exists on the acute management of aortic dissection, surgical treatment in ascending aorta dissection (type A) and medical treatment of descending aorta dissection (type B). In acute type B dissection, surgical or endovascular treament has usually been reserved for complications. In-hospital outcomes are generally acceptable in patients with uncomplicated acute type B dissection, up to 85–90% of whom survive to hospital discharge after receiving effective antihypertensive therapy [1]. However, a significant percentage who have successfully survived the acute phase with correct therapeutic management often require surgery during the chronic phase owing to aortic enlargement or, unfortunately, rupture of the aorta.

A. Evangelista, R. Aguilar, T. González-Alujas, P. Mahia, and J. Rodríguez-Palomares
Servei de Cardiología, Hospital Universitari Vall d'Hebron.

A. Evangelista (✉)
Servei de Cardiología, Hospital Universitari Vall d'Hebron,
P° Vall d'Hebron 119. 08035 Barcelona. Spain,
e-mail: aevangel@vhebron.net

Several studies have shown that the medium-to-long-term survival of treated patients with aortic dissection is 50–80% at 5 years and 30–60% at 10 years [2–8], regardless of the type of dissection, A or B [2, 9]. In patients with acute type A aortic dissection, surgical repair in the majority of patients is limited to the ascending aorta and, in some cases, additionally to the aortic arch. In De Bakey type I dissections, the aortic arch, and the downstream aorta remain dissected and are at risk for secondary dilatation in the near future. Eventhough surgery changes the natural history of type A aortic dissection, patients surviving surgical treatment may develop complications. These are basically associated with of surgical repair failure leading to progressive aortic root dilatation, with or without associated aortic regurgitation, or are secondary to persistent flow in the false lumen distal to the prosthetic tube.

Recent studies have shown follow-up mortality rates in patients discharged after acute type B aortic dissection to be relatively high, approaching 1 in 4 patients dying within 3 years [10]. Follow-up mortality after type B dissection exceeds that seen after acute type A aortic dissection and also exceeds the cumulative incidence of mortality in other diseases such as coronary artery disease or moderate chronic obstructive pulmonary disease [10]. It is considered that 31% to 66% of follow-up deaths are due to aorta-related complications such as rupture, extension of dissection and perioperative mortality from subsequent aortic or vascular repairs [6,10,11].

The advent of endovascular treatment, with lower morbidity and mortality than surgical treatment, raised new expectations for avoiding progressive enlargement and obtaining a complete remodelling of the aorta in the early management of non-complicated aortic dissection [12,13]. However, some patients with distal aortic dissection do not develop late aortic aneurysms and are succesfully managed for many years with medical treatment alone. Therefore, it is important to identify patients with a high risk of complications after the acute phase.

Predictors of Long-Term Aortic Dissection Evolution

Medical treatment after the acute phase is fundamental. Correct blood pressure control is associated with 96% survival free from aortic rupture at 5 years compared to 61% in the poorly-controlled group [14]. Suitable medical treatment with β-blockers is fundamental in preventing complications. β-blockers delay aortic dilatation by reducing blood pressure and dP/dt. The dose should be progressively increased until blood pressure is < 130/80 mm Hg.

Clinical Variables

Certain clinical predictive factors related to high risk of mortality during the long-term evolution of aortic dissection include age, chronic obstructive pulmonary disease, hypertension and Marfan syndrome [6,7,15]. Several studies have shown Marfan syndrome to be an independent predictor of late aneurysmal formation in descending aorta. After 5 years, only 50% of the Marfan patients presenting a residual dissection of the descending aorta remained complication-free or were surgically treated [6,7].

As in studies reporting in-hospital predictors of mortality, markers of malperfusion, kidney failure, hypotension and shock were significant independent predictors of death during follow-up in our study [3,5,16]. Therefore, although initial in-hospital management appeared to stabilise these severe hemodynamic and organ insults, we observed that such complications continued to have a negative impact on patient survival after discharge.

Finally, comorbidities such as atherosclerosis and a diseased aneurysmatic aorta have been shown in previous studies to predict in-hospital and follow-up outcomes [11]. Regarding a history of previous aortic aneurysm, pathology studies have suggested that the wall of an aneursymal aortic segment has decreased collagen synthesis, reduced elastin content and a thinner wall as part of a systemic problem [17,18]. These biophysical properties of the aorta predispose the entire aorta and its branches to dissection, further aneurysm formation and/or aortic rupture and may contribute to the high mortality rate in this group.

Imaging Variables

Advances in imaging techniques in the study of aortic disease provide new morphologic and dynamic information [19–21] that could be essential for predicting aortic dissection evolution and to identifying the subgroup of patients with a greater tendency to severe aortic enlargement.

Maximum Aortic Diameter

Maximum aortic dilatation in acute phase is a major predictor of complications during follow-up. Kato et al [22] showed that an aortic diameter > 40 mm in acute phase and a patent entry tear in the thoracic aorta were markers of an aneurysm developing in the false lumen (>60 mm) and that 80% of these patients required surgical reintervention at 5 years. A similar approach was considered by Marui et al [23]. Of 101 patients with type B dissection, 43 presented complications (diameter > 60 mm, an increasing diameter > 10 mm/year or aortic rupture) after a mean follow-up of 5 years. Only 6% of patients with maximum diameter < 40 mm and absence of flow in the false lumen evolved with complications versus 67% of patients with aortic diameter > 40 mm and flow in false lumen. Aneurysmal dilatation of the dissected aorta (Fig. 1) will occur in 25–40% of patients surviving acute type B aortic dissection [7,24]. Chronic dissecting type B aneurysms have a faster

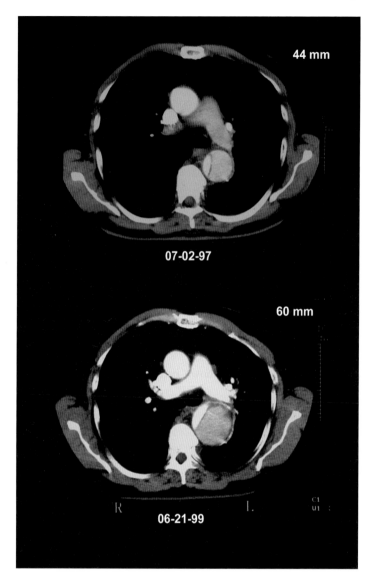

Fig. 1 Follow-up of type B dissection by CT showing 16mm aorta enlargement in 2 years. Note compression of the true lumen

expansion rate (3.7mm/y) compared to non-dissecting aneurysms (0.9mm/y), regardless of the initial size [25]. Secondary dilatation of the aorta during follow-up of aortic dissection has been considered a significant predictor of aortic rupture. Diameter > 60–65 mm [26] or annual growth > 4–5 mm [7,27] imply a high risk of aortic rupture, requiring consideration of surgical treatment.

Patent False Lumen

In addition to aortic diameter, a consistent predictor of outcomes in acute type B aortic dissection has been the hemodynamic status of the false lumen, classically divided into either a thrombosed false lumen or a patent false lumen. Studies have shown that completely thrombosed false lumens have improved outcomes, while patent false lumina have an increased risk of aortic expansion and death [9,21–23]. Persistence of patent false lumen in descending aorta is common in both dissection types and has been strongly associated with poor prognosis [9,22,23,27,28]. Total thrombosis of the false lumen, considered a precursor of spontaneous healing, is a rare event, even after surgical repair of a type A aortic dissections. A persistent false lumen can be found by TEE or MRI in most type B aortic dissection during follow-up and in more than 70% of type A aortic dissections after surgical repair [29]. Total thrombosis of the false lumen will progress to spontaneous healing of the aorta in only 4% of type III dissections. Persistent false lumen flow distal to the prosthetic tube cannot be considered a complication and long-term mortality and morbidity associated with this situation are high. After type A dissection repair, Ergin et al [30] observed that patent false lumen in descending aorta was linked to survival at 5 years of follow-up. Mortality in patients with patent false lumen was 37%, versus only 16% in those without patent false lumen in descending aorta. Thus, eliminating the entry port, and not just repairing the ascending aorta, is of great importance in surgical intervention.

Although several studies have shown patent false lumen to be a predictor of descending aorta dissection, the frequency of total false lumen thrombosis in the acute phase is 30–55% in the majority of series [22,23]. The high incidence of total false lumen thrombosis indicates that intramural hematomas, which have a different evolution pattern, were included in these studies [31].

Partial Thrombosis of False Lumen

Studies have shown that completely thrombosed false lumina have improved outcomes, while patent false lumina carry an increased risk of aortic expansion and death [21–23,32]. However, in the IRAD series (Fig. 2), partial thrombosis of the false lumen, defined as the concurrent presence of both flow and thrombus and present in a third of patients, was the strongest independent predictor of follow-up mortality with a 2.7-fold increased risk of death compared to patients with patent false lumen without thrombus formation [33].

Entry Tear Size

The prognostic value of entry tear size and a high false lumen pressure pattern has not been adequately analysed to date. TEE, CT and MRI permit a correct,

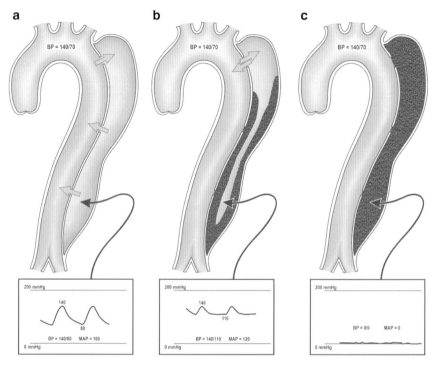

Fig. 2 Conceptual model of risk according to false lumen status. Panel (**a**) shows patent proximal and distal re-entry tears in absence of thrombus. Blood pressure tracing shows similar pressures in true and false lumina. Panel (**b**) shows patent entry tear and partial thrombosis forming a blind sac. Blood pressure tracing shows diastolic and mean arterial pressures in false lumen that exceed the pressure seen in panel (**a**). Panel (**c**) shows complete false lumen thrombosis with low blood pressure. From 33 with permission

on occasions complementary, assessment of entry tear size and location and false lumen hemokinetics. When the entry tear is small, the flow volume that enters the false lumen is low and thus the false lumen pressures will be low. When the entry tear is large (Fig. 3), the flow volume that enters the false lumen is large and diastolic pressures will be higher if there is no distal flow discharge through secondary communication tears or arterial trunk dissections [34]. The combination of a large entry tear and indirect signs of high pressure of the false lumen, distinguishable by imaging techniques, was the strong predictor of poor prognosis and related to higher mortality and aortic dilatation.

True Lumen Compression

Compression of the true lumen is an indirect sign of high pressure of the false lumen. Although true lumen compression is an easy variable to analyse [35], there

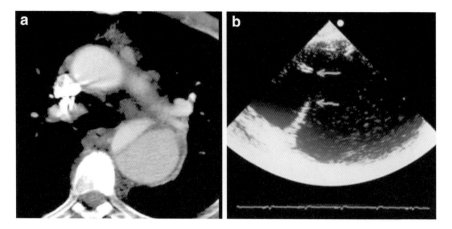

Fig. 3 (**a**) Computed tomography showing a type B dissection with large false lumen and compression of true lumen. (**b**) Large intimal tear in proximal part of descending aorta by transesophageal echocardiography

exist limitations secondary to local factors, as in spyroid dissection, that may determine decreases in true lumen size. Song et al [36] found that initial false lumen diameter at the upper thoracic aortic predicted late aneurysm with 100% sensitivity of and 76% specificity in their series. In this study the initial false lumen diameter (> 22 mm) was the most powerful predictor and was better than the initial aorta diameter in terms of predicting late aneurysmal change. A large false lumen probably reflects high false lumen pressure itself and generates an aorta aneurysm (Fig. 3). However, those studies had some limitations since both used CT, and intimal flap movement during the cardiac cycle was not considered. Low reproducibility of these measurements, spiral dissecction and lack of true lumen expansion after ascending aorta surgery are possible drawbacks to this finding.

Pathophysiological Mechanisms of Aortic Dilatation and Aortic Rupture.

Increase in wall tension secondary to enlargement of the aortic diameter or high false lumen pressure, as described by LaPlace's law, may elevate the risk of aneurysm expansion, re-dissection and rupture. Experimental studies have shown that a large entry tear and inadequate outflow from the false lumen may lead to a significant increase in mean arterial and diastolic pressure when compared to a lumen with adequate outflow despite similar systolic pressure [34,37,38]. On the other hand, in cases with similar entry tear size and distal communication, false lumen flow is rapid; however, when the entry tear is larger than distal communication, false lumen flow is slow and facilitates partial false lumen thrombosis. This

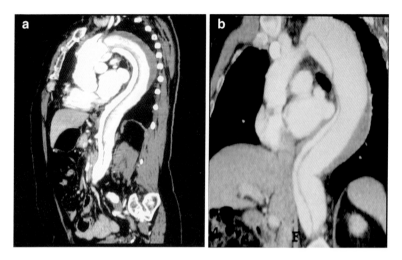

Fig. 4 Partial false lumen thrombosis in two different prognosis patterns of type B dissection. (**a**) Low-risk pattern with normal aorta size, small entry tear and no true lumen compression. (**b**) High-risk pattern with aortic enlargement, large entry tear and compression of the true lumen

mismatch or absence of distal discharge implies a higher diastolic pressure in false lumen that provokes greater enlargement or rupture of the false lumen. In fact, partial false lumen thrombosis is an epiphenomenon occurring more frequently when false lumen flow is slow, either because the entry tear is small or because the entry tear is large but without significant discharge. Although results in the literature are contradictory, partial thrombosis may be a predictor of good or poor prognosis depending on the size of the entry tear (Fig. 4). Another potential explanation lies in the understanding of partial thrombus formation which may occlude distal tears impeding outflow, and in the most extreme situation result in a blind sac [33]. Thus, a patient with partial thrombosis that impairs outflow from the false lumen may be at higher risk than a patient with adequate outflow from the false lumen via higher pressures and therefore wall tension.

Clinical Implications

The optimal treatment of descending aorta dissection remains under debate. Indications for stent grafting or surgery in the chronic phase are centred on the size and growth of the dissecting aneurysm. Complete proximal exclusion of the false lumen from the circulation has become the primary goal of endovascular stent therapy [38]. Treatment efficacy is greater in subacute phase than in chronic phase when the aorta is severely dilated and the intima less elastic. Since surgery on the descending aorta carries with significant peri-operative risks, the decision to operate is based on a delicate balance of the potential risk and benefits. Information from imaging techniques in the subacute phase of aortic dissection has significant prognostic value. In addition to maximum aorta diameter, which is associated with mortality and the need for surgical treatment during follow-up, a combination of entry tear size and image patterns consistent with high false lumen pressure is the best predictor of mortality and aortic dilatation, and surgical or endovascular treatment could be considered prior to discharge as the rate of progression of aortic dilatation is steeper shortly after the acute episode. On the other hand, patients without aortic dilatation and with small entry tear size have good prognosis and would be candidates for the established medical therapeutic management and standard clinical and imaging follow-up.

Follow-up with imaging techniques is essential to assess the appearance of a new dissection or aneurysm formation. The incidence of such recurrences can be around 25%, and some evolve with complications such as rupture and death by bleeding [39,40]. Careful follow-up is necessary to prevent the rupture of a dissecting aorta, and elective surgery should be considered if the aortic diameter exceeds 60 mm. Follow-up should include TEE or MRI before hospital discharge, an imaging procedure at 6 and 12 months and annually thereafter if the patient remains stable and asymptomatic.

References

1. Masuda Y, Yamada Z, Morooka N, et al (1991) Prognosis of patients with medically treated aortic dissections. Circulation 84:III7–13
2. Doroghazi RM, Slater EE, DeSanctis RW, et al (1984) Long-term survival of patients with treated aortic dissection. J Am Coll Cardiol 3:1026–34
3. Glower DD, Fann JI, Speier RH, et al (1990) Comparison of medical and surgical therapy for uncomplicated descending aortic dissection. Circulation. 82:IV39–46
4. Neya K, Omoto R, Kimura S, et al (1992) Outcome of standard type B acute aortic dissection. Circulation 86 (suppl II):II-1–7
5. Schor JS, Yerlioglu ME, Galla JD, et al (1996) Selective management of acute type B aortic dissection: long-term follow-up. Ann Thorac Surg 61:1339–41
6. Gysi J, Schaffner T, Mohacsi P, et al (1997) Early and late outcome of operated and non-operated acute dissection of the descending aorta. Eur J Cardiothorac Surg 11:1163–9; discussion 1169–70
7. Juvonen T, Ergin MA, Galla JD, et al (1999) Risk factors for rupture of chronic type B dissections. J Thorac Cardiovasc Surg 117:776–86
8. Estrera AL, Miller CC, Safi HJ, et al (2006) Outcomes of medical management of acute type B aortic dissection. Circulation 114 (suppl I):I-384–9
9. Bernard Y, Zimmermann H, Chocron S, et al (2001) False lumen patency as a predictor of late outcome in aortic dissection. Am J Cardiol 87:1378–82
10. Hagan PG, Nienaber CA, Isselbache EM, et al (2000) The International Registry of Acute Aortic Dissection. JAMA 283:897–903
11. Umaña JP, Lai DT, Mitchell RS, et al (2002) Is medical therapy still the optimal treatment strategy for patients with acute type B aortic dissections? J Thorac Cardiovasc Surg 124:896–910
12. Dake MD, Kato N, Mitchell RS, et al (1999) Endovascular stent-graft placement for the treatment of acute aortic dissection. N Engl J Med 340:1546–52

13. Nienaber CA, Fattori R, Lund G, et al (1999) Nonsurgical reconstruction of thoracic aortic dissection by stent-graft placement. N Engl J Med 340:1539–45
14. Nienaber CA, Eagle KA (2003) Aortic Dissection: New frontiers in diagnosis and management. Circulation 108:772–778
15. Yu H-Y, Chen Y-S, Huang S-C, et al (2004) Late outcome of patients with aortic dissection: study of a national database. Eur J Cardiothorac Surg:25:683.90
16. Suzuki T, Mehta RH, Ince H, et al (2003) Clinical profiles and outcomes of acute type B aortic dissection in the current era: lessons from the International Registry of Aortic Dissection. Circulation; 108 [suppl II]:II-312–7
17. Satta J, Laurila A, Paakko P, et al (1998) Chronic inflammation and elastic degradation in abdominal aortic aneurysm disease: an immunohistochemical and electron microscopic study. Eur J Vasc Endovasc Surg 15:313–9
18. Carmo M, Colombo L, Bruno A, et al (2002) Alteration of elastin, collagen and their crosslinks in abdominal aortic aneurysms. Eur J Vasc Endovasc Surg 23: 543–9
19. Strotzer M, Aebert H, Lenhart M, et al (2000) Morphology and hemodynamics in dissection of the descending aorta. Assessment with MR imaging. Radiology 41: 594–600
20. Yoshida S, Akiba H, Tamakawa N, et al (2003) Thoracic involvement of type A aortic dissection and intramural hematoma: diagnostic accuracy. Comparison of emergency helical CT and surgical findings. Radiology 228:430–5
21. Erbel R; Oelert H, Meyer J, et al (1993) Effects of medical and surgical therapy on aortic dissection evaluated by transesophageal echocardiography. Implications for prognosis and therapy. Circulation 87: 1604–15
22. Kato M, Bai H-z, Sato K, et al (1996) Determining surgical indications for acute type B dissection based on enlargement of aortic diameter during the chronic phase. Circulation 92 (suppleII): II-107–12
23. Marui A, Mochizuki T, Mitsui N, et al (1999) Toward the best treatment for uncomplicated patients with type B acute aortic dissection: A consideration for sound surgical indication. Circulation 100:II275–80
24. Elefteriades JA, Lovouolos CJ, Coady MA, et al (1999) Management of descending aortic dissection. Ann Thorac Surg 67:2002–5; discussion 2014–9
25. Coady MA, Rizzo JA, Hammond GL, et al (1999) Surgical intervention criteria for thoracic aortic aneurysms : a study of growth rates and complications. Ann Thorac Surg 67:1922–6
26. Hata M, Shiono M, Inoue T, et al (2003) Optimal treatment of type B acute aortic dissection: Long-term medical follow-up results. Ann Thorac Surg 75:1781–4
27. Onitsuka S, Akashi H, Tayama K, et al (2004) Long-term outcome and prognostic predictors of medically treated acute type B aortic dissections. Ann Thorac Surg 78:1268–73
28. Akutsu K, Nejima J, Kiuchi K, et al (2004) Effects of the patent false lumen on the long-term outcome of type B acute aortic dissection. Eur J Cardiothorac Surg 26:359–66
29. Mohr-Kahali S, erbel R, Rennollet H, et al (1989) Ambulatory follow-up of aortic dissection by transesophageal two-dimensional and color-coded Doppler echocardiography. Circulation 80:24–33
30. Ergin MA, Phillips RA, Galla JD, et al (1994) Significance of distal false lumen after type A dissection repair. Ann Thorac Surg 57:820–5
31. Evangelista A, Domínguez R, Sebastià C, et al (2003) Long-term follow-up of aortic intramural hematoma. Predictors of outcome. Circulation 108 583–9
32. Sueyoshi E, Sakamoto I, Hayashi K, et al (2004) Growth rate of aortic diameter in patients with type B aortic dissection during the chronic phase. Circulation110:II256–61
33. Tsai T, Evangelista A, Nienaber Ch, et al (2007) Partial trombosis of the lumen predicts follow-up death in patients with acute type B aortic dissection: a novel insight from the International Registry of Aortic Dissection. N Engl J Med 357:349–59
34. Chung JW, Elkins Ch, Sakai T, et al (2000) True-lumen collapse in aortic dissection. Part I. Evaluation of causative factors in phantoms with pulsatile flow. Radiology 214: 87–98
35. Immer FF, Krähenbühl E, Hagen U, et al (2005) Large area of the false lumen favors secondary dilatation of the aorta after acute type A aortic dissection. Circulation 112 (suppl I):I-49–52

36. Song JM, Kim SD, Kim JH, et al (2007) Long-term predictors of descending aorta aneurysmal change in patients with aortic dissection. J Am Coll Cardiol 50:799–804
37. Williams DM, Lee DY, Hamilton BH, et al (1997) The dissected aorta: part III. Anatomy and radiologic diagnosis of branch-vessel compromise. Radiology 203:37–44
38. Chung JW, Elkins Ch, Sakai T, et al (2000) True-lumen collapse in aortic dissection. Part II. Evaluation of treatment methods in phantoms with pulsatile flow. Radiology 214: 99–106
39. Nienaber Ch A, Zannetti S, Barbieri B, et al (2005) Investigation of stent graft in patients with type B aortic dissection: design of the INSTEAD trial a prospective, multicenter, European randomized trial. Am Heart J 149:592–9
40. Hsu R-B, Ho Y-L, Chen RJ, et al (2005) Outcome of medical and surgical treatment in patients with acute type B aortic dissection. Ann Thorac Surg 79:790–5

Symposium 2
Brain Protection in Aortic Arch Surgery

Spinal Cord Perfusion and Protection During Surgical and Endovascular Treatment of Descending Thoracic and Thoracoabdominal Aortic Aneurysms

Eva B. Griepp and Randall B. Griepp

Although the treatment in aortic surgery centers of carefully selected patients with thoracic and thoracoabdominal aortic aneurysms by surgical and endovascular techniques yields acceptable results, the fact remains that the majority of patients with extensive aneurysms are too frail for surgical resection, and cannot be treated by endovascular techniques because of the inability to revascularize aortic branches. Promising techniques for revascularizing the four abdominal branches (extra-anatomical debranching and branched grafts) are under development, but the problem of preserving spinal cord perfusion and viability remains a major roadblock.

It is our belief, however, that routine sacrifice of all intercostal and lumbar vessels is well within reach, and only awaits a more thorough understanding of spinal cord perfusion. To this end, we have carried out a number of experimental studies in a chronic pig model in which neurological function can be monitored intraoperatively, blood flow can be ascertained using microspheres, and outcome can be assessed in terms of behavioral recovery and histology.

In experiments involving crossclamping of the aorta, decreasing the body temperature from 37 to 32°C doubles the safe ischemic interval of the spinal cord, from 25 to 50 minutes, Fig. 1. Concomitant studies show that decreasing the body temperature from 37 to 32°C also halves the spinal cord blood flow. If a pig with intact segmental arteries is subjected to severe ischemia at normothermia, the spinal cord blood flow shows an immediate and dramatic hyperemic response upon release of the crossclamp, Fig. 2.

If all segmental vessels are sacrificed in the experimental situation–as may be required with open repair of extensive thoracoabdominal aneurysms, and will be inevitable if one wants to treat TAA/A with endografts–this does not result in loss of function, as reflected by motor evoked potentials (MEP), for at least an hour. Spinal cord perfusion pressure, which can be measured directly via a small catheter in a lower thoracic or upper lumbar segmental artery stump after it is detached from the aorta, falls to 20% of aortic pressure five hours after extensive segmental artery sacrifice; recovers to 60% of aortic pressure at 48 hours, and to 80% of aortic pressure

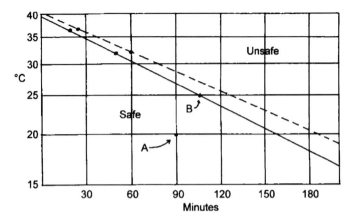

Fig. 1 This diagram is constructed from an experiments involving crossclamping of the aorta at normothermia and at 32C in pigs. The extrapolation from these experimental observations suggests the limits for safe ischemia of the spinal cord. Point A has been shown never to cause paraplegia in many experiments of prolonged slelective cerebral perfusion. Point B suggests the possible danger to the spinal cord of prolonged SCP at higher temperatures

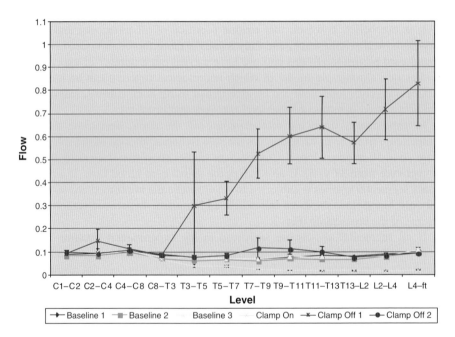

Fig. 2 This diagram is the result of data from a study of six pigs following aortic crossclamping for 20 minutes at normothermia: a severe ischemic insult, but one not likely to result in paraplegia. Microsphere-determined spinal cord blood flows are shown at the various levels along the spinal cord indicated along the horizonatal axis at baseline, immediately following aortic crossclamping; 5 minutes after release of the cross clamp, and one hour thereafter

Spinal Cord Perfusion and Protection

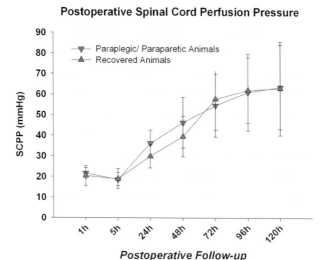

Fig. 3 Direct measurement of spinal cord perfusion pressures from a small catheter inserted into a low thoracic or high lumbar segmental vessel reveal a fall after segmental artery ligation which reaches its lowest point postoperatively. Even pigs that are paraplegic after extensive segmental artery ligation show recovery of spinal cord perfusion pressures to baseline within 72 hours. *From Etz CD, Homann TM, Plestis KA, Zhang N, Luehr M, Weisz DJ, Kleinman G, Griepp RB. Spinal cord perfusion after extensive segmental artery sacrifice: can paraplegia be prevented? Eur J Cardiothorac Surg 2007; 31:643–648, permission requested*

by 72 hours, Fig. 3. 50% of the pigs recover without neurological deficit, and 50% have some degree of spinal cord injury (paraplegia/paraparesis). Spinal cord blood flow, measured using microsphere techniques, never falls below hypothermic baseline values even in pigs that subsequently develop paraplegia. Pigs that sustain neurological injury differ from normal pigs only in that they do not mount a hyperemic response to warming and awakening 5 hours after SA ligation, Fig. 4.

Clinical studies confirm that many of the same observations regarding the response of the spinal cord circulation to sacrifice of segmental arteries can be made in patients undergoing extensive resection of thoracoabdominal aneurysms, Fig. 5. An increasing percentage of patients with spinal cord injury suffer delayed rather than immediate paraplegia, and these patients differ from controls in having a higher central venous pressures in the first few hours postoperatively, and a lower mean arterial pressure when compared to their normal ambulatory pressures (many have poorly controlled hypertension). Spinal cord perfusion pressures in patient show a drop an average of 2 hours after the last of the segmental arteries has been ligated, with a slow return to baseline values within 24 hours.

The explanation for these observations is in what we have termed the collateral network hypothesis of spinal cord perfusion. This understanding of spinal cord blood flow is buttressed by studies of casts of the vascular system in the pig (and similar studies carried out by others in humans), which show a very rich network

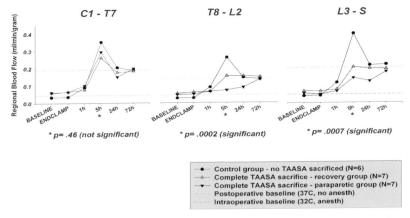

Fig. 4 When pigs that have undergone extensive ligation of segmental arteries (TAASA) are compared with pigs undergoing sham operations, at the time that pigs with TAASA ligation are experiencing a fall in spinal cord blood flow, those with intact TAASA show hyperemia. The dotted lines represent baseline spinal cord blood flows at 32C and at 37C. From Etz CD, Luehr M, Kari FA, Bodian CA, Smego D, Plestis KA, Griepp RB. Paraplegia after extensive thoracic and thoracoabdominal aortic aneurysm repair: Does critical spinal cord ischemia occur postoperatively? J Thorac Cardiovasc Surg 2008; in press, permission requested

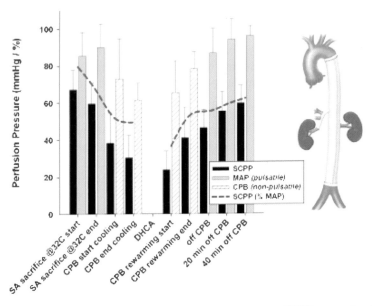

Fig. 5 If direct measurements of spinal cord perfusion pressures (SCPP) are undertaken in patients, a pattern of fall after segmental artery ligation is very similar to what is seen in experimental animals

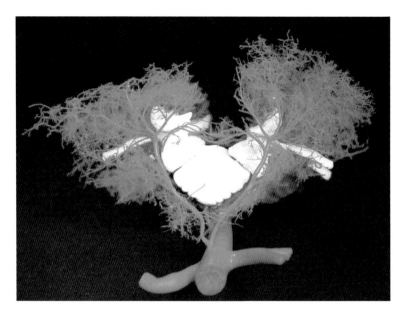

Fig. 6 A portion of a vascular cast from a pig, showing the extensive flow to paraspinal muscles from a lumbar segmental artery which can be seen arising from the aorta as a single branch, dividing into two lateral branches, which then contribute flow to the anterior spinal artery within the spinal canal. The two renal arteries can be seen arising from the aorta, as well as the vertebrae surrounding the spinal canal

Fig. 7 A frontal view of the anterior spinal artery from a vascular cast in a pig, showing what a tiny fragile vessel it is, and how minor a part of the dense collateral network surrounding the spinal cord

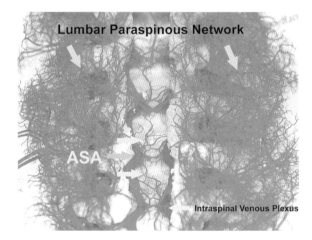

of vessels surrounding the spinal cord and the paraspinous muscles, Figs. 6 and 7. There is no single major contributor to the ASA, but multiple inputs, with significant flow from the segmental arteries, but also from the subclavian and hypogastric arteries. When the segmental arteries are sacrificed, the network of small arteries that nourishes the spinal cord is gradually reconstituted from the cranial and caudal

Fig. 8 Spinal cord blood flow studies using microspheres in the pig, demonstrating that flow to the spinal cord is only a small fraction of overall flow in the paraspinous collateral network, but that autoregulation allows its preservation following extensive segmental artery ligation

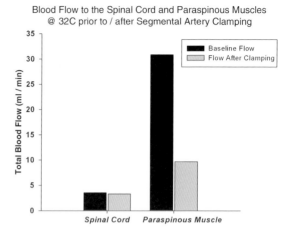

directions over a period of several days. With ischemia, blood flow to the muscles surrounding the spinal cord diminishes relatively more than the flow to the spinal cord, which is better preserved, Fig. 8.

There are a number of implications which arise from these observations with regard to avoiding spinal cord injury after surgical or endovascular treatment of extensive thoracic and thoracoabdominal aneurysms. Because of the very small absolute flow to the spinal cord from the collateral network, it is very important to avoid intraoperative steal. Any source of intraoperative ischemia must be avoided because it may provoke a need not only for baseline flow postoperatively, but for spinal cord hyperemia: thus distal perfusion is critical during open repair. Reduction of spinal cord metabolism using mild hypothermia is a very important safeguard. Preservation of inflow from the subclavian and hypogastric arteries is also critical.

The role of a high mean arterial pressure is important not only intraoperatively, but for at least 24 hours after segmental artery ligation, since the lowest levels of spinal cord perfusion pressure are seen a few hours postoperatively, and pressures do not return to normothermic baseline values for many hours after surgery. During this vulnerable interval, protecting the spinal cord from injury involves monitoring function by means of somatosensory evoked potentials; keeping central venous pressures low, and draining cerebrospinal fluid to avoid impeding spinal cord perfusion. Obvious threats to spinal cord perfusion such as fever and bleeding must of course also be avoided.

These findings suggest that hemodynamic and metabolic manipulations lasting only 48 to 72 hours should enable routine sacrifice of all segmental vessels without spinal cord injury, making endovascular treatment of the entire thoracoabdominal aorta a foreseeable possibility.

Selected References

Etz CD, Homann TM, Plestis KA, et al (2007) Spinal cord perfusion after extensive segmental artery sacrifice: can paraplegia be prevented? Eur J Cardiothorac Surg 31:643–648

Etz CD, Halstead JC, Spielvogel D, et al (2006) Thoracic and thoracoabdominal aneurysm repair: is reimplantation of spinal cord arteries a waste of time? Ann Thorac Surg 82:1670–1677

Etz CD, Homann TM, Plestis KA, et al (2007) Spinal cord perfusion after extensive segmental artery sacrifice: can paraplegia be prevented? Eur J Cardiothorac Surg 31:643–8

Etz CD, Luehr M, Kari FA, et al (2008) Paraplegia after extensive thoracic and thoracoabdominal aortic aneurysm repair: Does critical spinal cord ischemia occur postoperatively? J Thorac Cardiovasc Surg (in press)

Griepp RB, Griepp EB (2007) Spinal cord perfusion and protection during descending thoracic and thoracoabdominal aortic surgery: the collateral network concept. Ann Thorac Surg 83:S865–S869; discussion S890–S892.

Halstead JC, Wurm M, Etz C, et al (2007) Preservation of spinal cord function after extensive segmental artery sacrifice: regional variations in perfusion. Ann Thorac Surg 84:789–794

Strauch JT, Spielvogel D, Lauten S, et al (2003) Importance of extrasegmental vessels for spinal cord blood supply in a chronic porcine model. Eur J Cardiothorac Surg 24:817–824

Strauch JT, Lauten A, Spielvogel D, et al (2004) Mild hypothermia protects the spinal cord from ischemic injury in a chronic porcine model. Eur J Cardiothorac Surg 25:708–715

Brain Protection in Aortic Arch Surgery

Eva B. Griepp and Randall B. Griepp

Protection of the brain during aortic arch surgery has been– and continues to be– the primary consideration in carrying out these complex operations. Cerebral damage occurs primarily due to two mechanisms: global injury secondary to inadequate protection of the brain during interruptions of normal cerebral perfusion, and focal defects resulting from embolization of atheroma and surgical debris into the cerebral vessels. If techniques for cerebral protection are to improve, an integrated approach to address both mechanisms of injury will be required.

Hypothermia is the mainstay of essentially all techniques of global cerebral protection. The principal benefit of hypothermia is a reduction in cerebral metabolic demands. As seen in Fig. 1, cerebral metabolism is reduced 50% when the temperature is reduced to 28°C, and to 19% of its normothermic value at 18°C. If one assumes that cerebral ischemia at normothermia can be tolerated without injury for 5 minutes, then hypothermic circulatory arrest (HCA) at 18°C is theoretically safe for only 25 minutes. In fact, laboratory investigations as well as clinical studies of cognitive function and the incidence of temporary neurological dysfunction strongly suggest that intervals of hypothermic circulatory arrest (HCA) longer than 30 minutes even at esophageal temperatures of 13–15°C may be associated with cerebral injury.

In the hope of improving cerebral protection and perhaps flushing out embolic debris, the use of retrograde cerebral perfusion (RCP)–infusion of cold blood into the superior vena cava–was initially greeted with enthusiasm. Introduced by Ueda and still felt by many to be a useful cerebral protective technique, RCP has been abandoned in our institution based on laboratory studies and analysis of our clinical outcomes. Selective cerebral perfusion (SCP), introduced by Kazui and Bachet, has proven to be superior both to HCA alone and to HCA combined with RCP. For intervals of interruption of normal cerebral perfusion for more than 30 minutes, we believe it to be the technique of choice.

Optimal parameters for the application of SCP are still being evaluated both clinically and in the experimental animal. In a series of experiments in the pig in

E.B. Griepp and R.B. Griepp
Department of Cardiothoracic Surgery, The Mount Sinai School of Medicine,
One Gustav Levy Place, New York, NY, USA

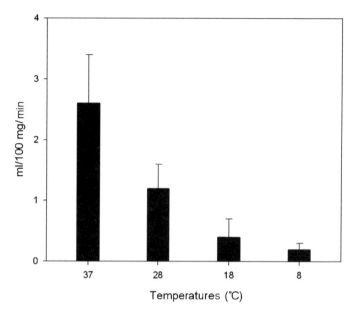

Fig. 1 Cerebral metabolism at various hypothermic temperatures in juvenile Yorkshire pigs. *From Ehrlich MP, McCullough JN, Zhang N, Weisz DJ, Juvonen T, Bodian CA, Griepp RB. Effect of hypothermia on cerebral blood flow and metabolism in the pig. Ann Thorac Surg 2002; 73:191–7. permission requested*

which cerebral oxygen consumption and cerebral blood flow were measured, and functional behavioral outcome was used as the assay, we have made a number of potentially useful observations. SCP flow that generates a perfusion pressure of 50 to 70 mmHg results in better functional outcome than SCP with a higher pressure, perhaps reflecting the fact that high pressure perfusion results in an inappropriate rise in oxygen consumption after SCP, Fig. 2. Temperatures of 10–15°C result in more effective and sustained reduction of metabolism during SCP and recovery, Fig. 3, and therefore in a better behavioral outcome than temperatures from 20–25°C, Fig. 4. A hematocrit of 30% is associated with flow rates significantly lower during SCP than a hematocrit of 20%, Fig. 5, but results in superior behavioral outcome. pH-stat acid-base management, although providing a higher cerebral blood flow, Fig. 6, does not confer any outcome benefit over perfusion using alpha-stat principles in healthy pigs. Others have suggested that in dogs with a previous cerebral infarct, pH-stat management may be beneficial.

But whether all these findings are directly translatable to the clinical setting is not certain. In principle, it seems reasonable to favor perfusion parameters associated with lower flow rates—and therefore a lower risk of embolization—if the outcomes are the same. Recent clinical series are focusing on whether SCP can be carried out safely at higher temperatures. Careful analysis will be necessary to

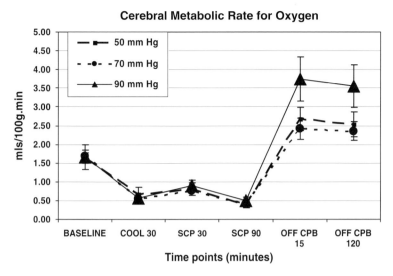

Fig. 2 Cerebral metabolism following 90 minutes of selective cerebral perfusion at various pressures in Yorkshire pigs. *From Halstead JC, Meier M, Wurm M, Ning Zhang N, Spielvogel D, Weisz D, Bodian C, Griepp RB. Optimizing selective cerebral perfusion: deleterious effects of high perfusion pressures. J Thorac Cardiovasc Surg, in press, permission requested*

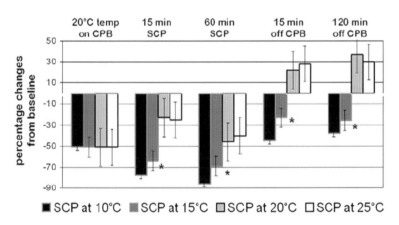

Fig. 3 Cerebral metabolism during and following selective cerebral perfusion (SCP) at various temperatures in juvenile Yorkshire pigs, compared with baseline normothermic values. * indicates a significant difference between values at 10–15C vs 20–25C. *From Strauch JT, Spielvogel D, Lauten A, Zhang N, Rinke S, Weisz D, Bodian CA, Griepp RB. Optimal temperature for selective cerebral perfusion. J Thorac Cardiovasc Surg 2005: 130:75–82, permission requested*

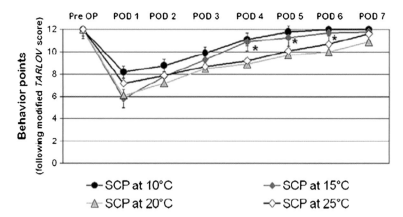

Fig. 4 Behavioral outcome following SCP at different temperatures during SCP in same experiment as in Figure 3. A behavioral score of 12 indicates normal recovery of function. POD, postoperative day; * indicates a significant difference between groups at 10–15C and 20–25C. From Strauch et al, as in Figure 3, permission requested

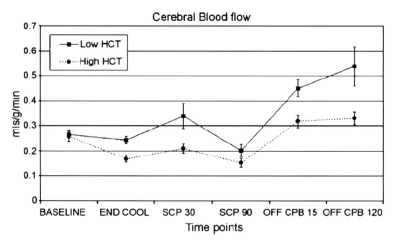

Fig. 5 Cerebral blood flow during and following SCP in Yorkshire pigs at hematocrits of 20% and 30%. From Halstead JC, Wurm M, Meier DM, Zhang N, Spielvogel D, Weisz D, Bodian C, Griepp RB. Avoidance of hemodilution during selective cerebral perfusion enhances neurobehavioural outcome in a survival porcine model. Eur J Cardiothorac Surg 2007; 32:518–520, permission requested

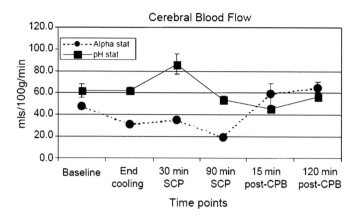

Fig. 6 Cerebral blood flow during and following SCP in Yorkshire pigs using pH stat and alpha-stat management of acid-base balance during cooling, SCP and rewarming. *From Halstead JC, Spielvogel D, Meier DM, Weisz D, Bodian C, Griepp RB. Optimal pH strategy for selective cerebral perfusion. Eur J Cardiothorac Surg 2005; 28:266–273, discussion 273, permission requested*

ascertain whether cerebral as well as lower body organ preservation is equivalent or better than with hypothermic perfusion, and whether advantages of better hemostasis are demonstrable.

Focal embolic injury depends primarily on surgical technique. It is imperative to avoid dislodgement of atheroma or clot into the cerebral circulation before opening any cerebral vessels, and to remove any surgical debris from cerebral vessels prior to reinstitution of perfusion. Particularly in patients with atherosclerotic aneurysms, we believe that avoidance of embolic injury requires cannulation remote from the aortic arch, with no extensive atheromatous disease present between the cannulation site and the cerebral vessels. In our view, axillary artery perfusion is superior to both aortic and femoral cannulation.

Dissection of diseased cerebral vessels can most safely be carried out during a period of HCA, and anastomoses should be constructed beyond major atheromatous disease. The introduction of branched grafts–primarily in Japan–has been a major advance in this area. We currently believe that using a trifurcation graft with a separate anastomosis to the arch is the optimal technique: in cases of complex arch disease, it allows flexibility in the cerebral vessel implantation site as well in choosing the site of the elephant trunk anastomosis, as shown in Fig. 7.

Cerebral protection has advanced quite substantially over the past decade. In major centers, arch resection is routinely being accomplished with mortality and stroke rates of less than 5%.

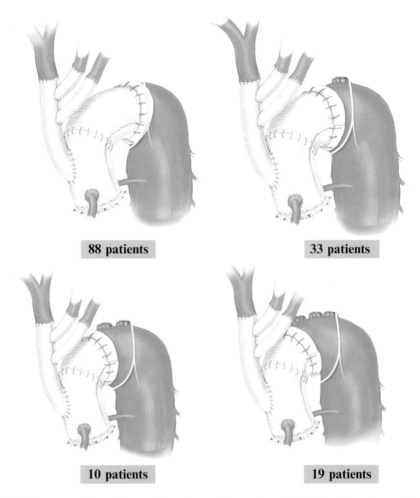

Fig. 7 Diagrams of the various configurations which can be used with the trifurcation graft for aortic arch reconstructions, with the numbers of patients in which each variation was utilized in our recent experience. *From Spielvogel D, Etz CD, Silovitz D, Lansman SL, Griepp RB. Aortic arch replacement with a trifurcated graft. Ann Thorac Surg 2007; 83:S791–S795; discussion S824–S831, permission requested*

Selected References

Bachet J, Guilmet D (2002) Brain protection during surgery of the aortic arch. J Card Surg 17:115–24

Ehrlich MP, Hagl C, McCullough JN, et al (2001) Retrograde cerebral perfusion provides negligible flow through brain capillaries in the pig. J Thorac Cardiovasc Surg 122:331–8

Ehrlich MP, McCullough JN, Zhang N, et al (2002) Effect of hypothermia on cerebral blood flow and metabolism in the pig. Ann Thorac Surg 73:191–7

Halstead JC, Spielvogel D, Meier DM, et al (2005) Optimal pH strategy for selective cerebral perfusion. Eur J Cardiothorac Surg 28:266–273, discussion 273

Etz CD, Plestis KA, Silovitz D, et al (2008) Axillary cannulation significantly improves survival and neurological outcome after atherosclerotic aneurysm repair of the aortic root and ascending aorta. Ann Thorac Surg (in press)

Halstead JC, Etz C, Meier M, et al (2007) Perfusing the cold brain: optimal neuroprotection for aortic surgery. Ann Thorac Surg 84:768–774; discussion 774

Halstead JC, Meier M, Wurm M, et al (2008) Optimizing selective cerebral perfusion: deleterious effects of high perfusion pressures. J Thorac Cardiovasc Surg, in press

Halstead JC, Wurm M, Meier DM, et al (2007) Avoidance of hemodilution during selective cerebral perfusion enhances neurobehavioural outcome in a survival porcine model. Eur J Cardiothorac Surg 32:518–520

Kamiya H, Hagl C, Kropivnitskaya I, et al (2007) The safety of moderate hypothermic lower body circulatory arrest with selective cerebral perfusion: a propensity score analysis. J Thorac Cardiovasc Surg 133:501–9

Kazui T (2007) Normothermic selective cerebral perfusion – how safe it is? Eur J Cardiothorac Surg

Kazui T, Yamashita K, Washiyama N, et al (2007) Aortic arch replacement using selective cerebral perfusion. Ann Thorac Surg 83:S796–8; discussion S824–31

Spielvogel D, Halstead JC, Meier M, et al (2005) Aortic arch replacement using a trifurcated graft: simple, versatile and safe. Ann Thorac Surg 80:90–95; discussion 95

Spielvogel D, Etz CD, Silovitz D, et al (2007) Aortic arch replacement with a trifurcated graft. Ann Thorac Surg 83:S791–S795; discussion S824–S831

Strauch JT, Spielvogel D, Lauten A, et al (2005) Optimal temperature for selective cerebral perfusion. J Thorac Cardiovasc Surg 130:75–82

Strauch JT, Spielvogel D, Lauten A, et al (2004) Axillary artery cannulation: routine use in ascending aorta and aortic arch replacement. Ann Thorac Surg 78:103–108; discussion 108

Strauch JT, Spielvogel D, Lauten A, et al (2004) Technical advances in total aortic arch replacement. Ann Thorac Surg 77:581–589; discussion 589–590

Ueda Y, Miki S, Kusuhara K, et al (1990) Surgical treatment of aneurysm or dissection involving the ascending aorta and aortic arch, utilizing circulatory arrest and retrograde cerebral perfusion. J Cardiovasc Surg 31:553–8

Tools and Tricks in Monitoring the Brain During Arch Surgery

Marc Schepens

While performing aortic arch surgery, it is mandatory to rely on a safe neuroprotective strategy to avoid cerebral damage, the most dreadful complication after repair of the arch. This can only be achieved by a combination of different modalities.

Moderate (25 degrees Celsius rectal temperature) to deep (18 degrees Celsius or lower rectal temperature) cooling of the body during extracorporeal circulation is a cornerstone as well as the antegrade cerebral perfusion, the latter especially in complex arch reconstructions. While time limits the use of deep hypothermic circulatory arrest to about 30 minutes, there are almost no time restrictions when using antegrade selective cerebral perfusion.

Continuous bilateral radial artery pressure monitoring is an easy and cheap way to have some information about the blood flow in the arch. This technique can be applied in almost every patient.

Continuous electroencephalography gives useful information about regional disturbances in cerebral blood flow but can also be used in conjunction with the technique of deep hypothermic circulatory arrest. It gives only information about the cortical areas of the brain.

Bilateral transcranial doppler monitoring of the blood flow in both middle cerebral arteries gives very useful information about the cerebral blood flow. This technique is advisable during antegrade selective cerebral perfusion to control the blood flow in both cerebral hemispheres. It gives also information about e.g. kinking of the catheters and microembolic particles such as air, debris, calcium, clots. It is a time-consuming procedure and it requires a long-lasting monitoring session during surgery.

Bilateral near infrared spectroscopy is a noninvasive, non-expensive and reproducible bedside technique that gives information about the oxygenation of the frontal lobes of the brain. Cerebral blood flow cannot be measured quantitatively.

Of course all the above-mentioned techniques cannot always be applied simultaneously since some of them are dependent of skilled and trained personnel which is not always available 24 hours a day. Surgeons and anesthesiologists should at least try to incorporate maximal safety provisions to protect maximally the central neurologic functions of their patients.

M. Schepens (✉)
AZ St. Jan, Brugge, Belgium

Brain Protection in Aortic Surgery–Antegrade Selective Cerebral Perfusion

Teruhisa Kazui

Summary It is critical to select the appropriate strategy for protecting the brain from ischemic and embolic injury during arch operation. Our current strategy for protecting the brain from ischemic injury is that antegrade selective cerebral perfusion (SCP) is the method of choice if cerebral protection time to be required exceeds 30 minutes.

Moderately hypothermic two-vessel (innominate artery (IA) or right axillary artery (RAxA) and left commen carotid artery (LCCA)) is safe and effective for brain protection in a majority of the patients. Three-arch vessel (IA or RAxA, LCCA and left subclavian artery (LSA)) or one-arch vessel (RAxA) is used in selected patients on the basis of presence or absence of intra- and extra-cranial arterial disease, expected duration of cerebral protection and extent of aortic replacement. As for protecting the brain from embolic injury, it is important to select the appropriate cannulation site for instituting cardiopulmonary bypass and antegrade SCP and operative technique of arch repair.

By the end of March, 2007, 500 patients underwent arch repair using antegrade SCP. The over–all in hospital mortality, permanent and temporary neurological dysfunction were 4.0 %, 3.2 %, and 4.4 %, respectively in recent 294 patients even with inclusion of emergency cases.

Keywords cerebral protection · antegrade SCP · two-arch vessel perfusion · total arch replacement · cerebral embolism

T. Kazui (✉)
Cardiovascular Center Hokkaido Ohno Hospital, 4-1-1-30 Nishino,
Nishi-ku, Sapporo, Hokkaido, Japan 063-0034
e-mail: tkazui@cvc-ohno.or.jp

Introduction

On the basis of experimental and clinical studies, our current strategy for cerebral protection is as follows; Deep hypothermic circulatory arrest (DHCA) with or without retrograde cerebral perfusion (RCP) is applied to the selected cases in which the expected cerebral protection time is less than 30 minutes, which is now considered to be the safe duration of cerebral protection. On the other hand, SCP is exclusively used for cases requiring longer cerebral protection time such as total arch replacement which usually requires 60–90 miniutes in our hand.

This chapter elucidates the technique of antegrade SCP during moderate hypothermic circulatory arrest in patients undergoing aortic arch repair.

History of Antegrade SCP

Looking at the history of antegrade SCP, which is longer than that of RCP, in 1957, Dr. DeBakey and collegues first applied SCP as a cerebral protection method in arch aneurysm surgery[1]. But the normothermic high flow and high pressure SCP resulted in a rather high incidence of cerebral complication. The technique was, therefore, abandoned after that.

Since then, several authors including Dr. Bloodwell [2], Dr. Pearce [3], Dr. Crawford [4], Dr. Cooley [5], Dr. Frist [6], our group [7], Dr. Bachet [8], Dr. Baribeau [9], Dr. Tasdemir [10], Dr. Touati [11] have reported their own modification of SCP including perfusion sites, volume, pressure, and temperature etc (Table 1). Since the optimum details of the perfusion technique have not been established, the results obtained with these techniques have varied widely in the literature.

Table 1 History of antegrade selective cerebral perfusion

Antegrade Selective Cerebral Perfusion					
Year	Author	Perfusion site	Temp.	Flow/Pressure	Pump head
1957	DeBakey	IA + LCCA	norm	high	one
1966	Bloodwell	IA + LCCA + LAxA	norm	high	three
1969	Pearce	RBA + LCCA + LBA	norm	high	one
1979	Crawford	IA + LCCA	norm	low (65–100 mmHG)	one
1981	Cooley	IA + LCCA	moderate (24~26°C)	low	one
1986	Frist	IA or LCCA	moderate (26~28°C)	low	one
1989	Kazui	IA + LCCA	moderate (22~25°C)	low	one
1991	Bachet	IA + LCCA	deep (6~12°C)	low	one
1998	Baribeau	RAxA	moderate (22°C)	low	one
2002	Tasdemir	RBA	moderate (26°C)	low	one
2006	Touati	IA + LCCA	norm	low	one

IA: innominate artery, LCCA: left common carotid artery, LAxA: left axillary artery, RBA: right brachial artery, LBA: left brachial artery, norm: normothermia

In 1986, we modified this technique to a moderately hypothermic, low flow and low pressure perfusion.

Cardiopumonary Bypass

Cardiopulmonary bypass (CPB) is established by cannulating the ascending aorta or RAxA, when necessary, for arterial inflow, and the right atrium using a single two-staged cannula for venous drainage. After CPB is established, the left ventricular vent is inserted through the right superior pulmonary vein. Myocardial protection is provided by both antegrade and retrograde blood cardioplegia. Epiaortic echo scanning and transesophageal echocardiography are routinely performed to select the site of arterial cannulation.

If the ascending aorta is free from atherosclerotic debris, it is preferred site for arterial cannulation. If the ascending aoeta is found to be inappropriate because of the presence of atherosclerotic debris, the alternative site for arterial cannulation is RAxA. An 8-mm Dacron graft is sutured to this artery in an end-to-side fashion.

Antegrade SCP Protocol

In principle, the bilateral two-arch vessel perfusion technique is sed (Fig. 1) [12,13].

Both IA and LCCA are perfused at a rate of 10 ml/kg/min at a rectal temperature of 25°C by a single pump separate from the systemic circulation. LSA is kept cross-clamped during SCP. The right radial arterial pressure as well as the bilateral catheter tip pressure is adjusted at around 40 mmHg to regulate the perfusion pressure. Arterial blood pH is managed according to the α-stat strategy during CPB.

If RAxA is used for arterial cannulation, systemic perfusion is started through the graft sutured to this artery together with the femoral artery and after cooling the patient, IA is cross- clamped proximally, LCCA is cannulated, and both RAxA and LCCA are perfused as SCP (Fig. 2).

Three-arch vessel perfusion, that is, additional LSA perfusion is performed in selected patients, who have occlusion of right vertebral artery, dominant left vertebral artery, and lack of efficient intracranial arterial communication to avoid the risk of vertebrobasilar artery insufficiency.

More recently, unilateral cerebral perfusion through RAxA instead of the bilateral cerebral perfusion is used in selected patients who undergo hemiarch replacement requiring rather short period of cerebral protection (Fig. 3). CPB is initiated through RAxA and femoral arteries. After cooling down to a rectal temperature of 20°C, both IA and LCCA are cross-clamped at their origins, and systemic circulatory arrest is induced. The unilateral cerebral perfusion through RAxA is maintained at a rate of 10/ml/kg/min.

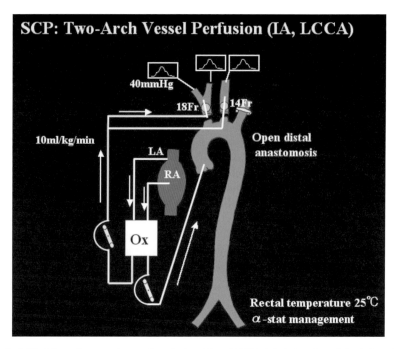

Fig. 1 SCP: Bilateral two-arch vessel perfusion (IA + LCCA) LA: left atrium, RA: right atrium, Ox: oxygenator

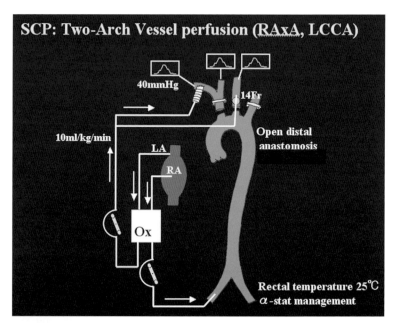

Fig. 2 SCP: Bilateral two-arch vessel perfusion (RAxA + LCCA) LA: left atrium, RA: right atrium, Ox: oxygenator

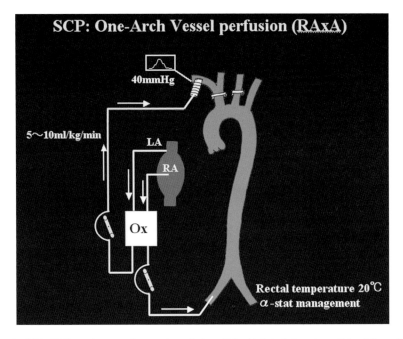

Fig. 3 SCP: Unilateral one-arch vessel perfusion (RAxA) LA: left atrium, RA: right atrium, Ox: oxygenator

Advantages of Antegrade SCP

Antegrade SCP presents several advantages when compared to DHCA with or without RCP. They are; 1) it can extend the safe duration of cerebral protection up to 90 minutes, and facilitates complex aortic arch repair. 2) it obviates the need of deep hypothermia thus reducing the pump time, and the risk of hypothermia-related complications such as pulmonary insufficiency and coagulopathy. 3) SCP is more effective in supplying oxygenated blood to the brain resulting in more physiological brain energy metabolism, and thus is the most reliable method of brain protection.

Operative Technique of Arch Repair

The selection of operative technique of arch repair is also important. Two different kinds of operative technique have been used. One is hemiarch or partial arch replacement and other is total arch replacement. The latter includes the en bloc or island technique and the separated graft technique. Figure 4 shows the separated graft technique which is now our preferred surgical technique [14,15]. Under SCP with systemic circulatory arrest, the distal end of the arch graft is sutured to the descending aortic stump. Antegrade perfusion is started from the side branch of the arch graft. The LSA is sutured to the third branch of the arch graft. Then rewarming

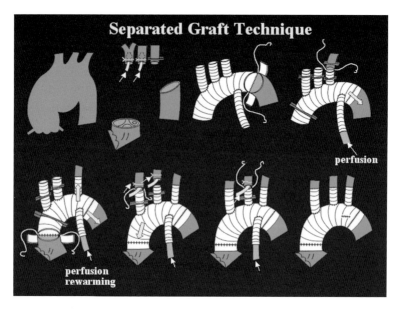

Fig. 4 Separated graft technique using 4-branched aortic arch graft

by CPB is started. The proximal end of the arch graft is sutured to the ascending aortic stump. The coronary circulation is started after deairing the graft. Then the IA and LCCA are sutured to the corresponding branches of the arch graft.

Advantages of Separated Graft Technique

Separated graft technique presents several advantages over the en bloc or island technique in which the arch vessels are reimplanted to the side hole of the graft [16]. They include: 1) arch vessel anastomoses are performed at the intact distal arteries where they are free from atherosclerotic debris or dissection, 2) pathological portion of the aortic arch can be completely resected in a Marfan's patient, 3) bleeding from the site of the arch vessel anastomoses can be easily controlled, 4) antegrade systemic perfusion through the arch graft prevents the retrograde embolization or organ malperfusion, and 5) total pump time and systemic circulatory arrest time are shorter than those in the en bloc technique.

Protection of Brain Embolism

It has been indicated that permanent neurological dysfunction usually results from cerebral emboli, and seems to have nothing to do with the cerebral protection method, although suboptimal cerebral protection obviously will aggravates focal injury.

Therefore, it is critical to protect the brain from embolic injury during the operation. The measures we have taken for this are; 1) epiaortic echo scanning on the ascending aorta to select the site of arterial cannulation, 2) RAxA cannulation if the ascending aorta is not suitable for cannulation, 3) distal intact arch vessel cannulation to avoid the dislogement of atheroma during cannulation, 4) antegrade systemic perfusion after the distal graft anastomosis to reduce the risk of distal embolization, and 5) complete resection of the aorta containing the clot or atheroma using the separated graft technique.

Results

Five hundred patients underwent surgery for arch aneurysm or dissection using hypothermic CPB and antegrade SCP until the end of March 2007. The patient's mean age was 65 ranging from 18 to 92, and 65% of them were male. Etiologies of the aortic disease were acute dissection in 27% of the patients, chronic dissection in 21%, and non-dissection in 52%.

Emergency operation was performed in 29% of the patients for rupture of aneurysm or acute aortic dissection.

Number of arch vessels useed for SCP were two-vessel in 91% of the patients, single-vessel in 6% and three-vessel in 3%.

As for the extent of aortic replacement, patch angioplasty was used in only 1% of the patients performed in earlier period. Graft replacement was performed in the remaining 99% of the patients; ascending and hemiarch replacement in 12%, ascending and total arch replacement in 36%, isolated total arch replacement in 2%, total arch and desending aortic replacement in 2%, and ascending, total arch, and descending aortic replacement in 47%. Overall total arch replacement was performed in 437 patients (87%), and simultaneous descending aortic replacement in 49% of the patients. Two hundred sixty four concomitant procedures were performed including elephant trunk procedure, AVR, CABG, aortic valve resuspension, mitral valve or replacement, and abdominal aneurysm repair.

The overall in-hospital mortality was 9.0%, but it significantly decreased to 4.0% in the recent 294 patients operated on since 1997, including the emergency cases.

The overall postoperative temporary and permanent neurological dysfunction were 4.4% and 3.2%, respectively. No significant difference was noted between the two different operative periods.

Mean SCP time was 87 minutes in the late series. There was no significant correlation between SCP time and in-hospital mortality or postoperative neurological dysfunction.

References

1. DeBakey ME, Crawford ES, Cooley DA, et al (1957) Successful resection of fusiform aneurysm of aortic arch with replacement by homograft. Sur Gynecol Obstet 105:657–664

2. Bloodwell RD, Hallman GL, Cooley DA (1968) Total replacement of the aortic arch and the subclavin steal phenomenon. Ann Thorac Surg 5:236–245
3. Pearce CW, Wechert RF 3rd, del Real RE (1969) Aneurysm of the aortic arch. Simplified technique for excision and prosthetic Replacement (1969) 58:886–890
4. Crawford ES, Saleh SA, Schuessler JS (1979) Treatment of aneurysm of transverse aortic arch. J Thorac Cardiovasc Surg 78:383–393
5. Cooley DA, Ott D, Fraizer OH, et al (1981) Surgical treatment of aneurysm of the tranverse aortic arch: experience with 25 patients using hypothermic techniques. Ann Thorac Surg 32:260–272
6. Frist WH, Baldwin JC, Starnes VA, et al (1986) A reconsideration of cerebral perfusion in aortic arch replacement. Ann Thorac Surg 42:273–281
7. Kazui T, Inoue N, Komatsu S (1989) Surgical treatment of aneurysmof the transverse aortic arch. J Cardiovasc Surg 30:402–406
8. Bachet J, Guilmet D, Goudot B, et al (1991) A new technique of cerebral protection during operations on the transverse aortic arch. J Thorac Cardiovasc Surg 102:85–93
9. Baribeau, YR, Westbrook, BM, Charlesworth, DC, et al (1998) Arterial inflow via an axillary artery graft for the severely atheromatous aorta. Ann Thorac Surg 66:33–37
10. Tasdemir O, Saritas A, Kucuker S, et al (2002) Aortic arch repair with right brachial artery perfusion. Ann Thorac Surg 73:1837–1842
11. Touati GD, Marticho P, Farag M, et al (2007) Totally normothermic aortic arch replacement without circulatory arrest. Eur J Cardiothorac Surg 32:263–268
12. Kazui T, Inoue N, Yamada O, et al (1992) Selective cerebral perfusion during operation for aneurysms of the aortic arch: a reassessment. Ann Thorc Surg 53:109–114
13. Kazui T, Kimura N, Yamada O, et al (1994) Surgical outcome of aortic arch aneurysms using selective cerebral perfusion. Ann Thorc Surg 57:904–911
14. Kazui T, Washiyama N, Bashar AHM, et al (2000) Total arch replacement using aortic arch branched grafts with the aid of antegrade selective cerebral perfusion. Ann Thorc Surg 70:3–9
15. Kazui T, Washiyama N, Bashar AHM, et al (2001) Improved results of atherosclerotic arch aneurysm operations with a refined technique. J Thorac Cardiovasc Surg 121:491–499
16. Di Eusanio M, Schepens MA, Morishuis WJ, et al (2004) Separate grafts or en bloc anastomosis for arch vessels reimplantation to the aortic arch. Ann Thorac Surg 77:2021–2028

Intermittent Pressure Augmented Retrograde Cerebral Perfusion

Shinichi Takamoto, Kan Nawata, Tetsuro Morota, Kazuo Kitahori, and Mitsuhiro Kawata

Having an experimental finding that intermittent pressure augmented RCP (IPA-RCP) significantly reduced postoperative brain damage in a canine model, we utilize IPA-RCP in clinical settings. IPA-RCP requires intermittent augmentation of superior vena caval pressure up to 45 mmHg every thirty seconds, while conventional RCP (C-RCP) continuous pressure of 15 mmHg. We examined the impact of IPA-RCP on the outcome of aortic arch surgery. Methods Since January 1999, we have had seventy-seven operations of total arch replacement via midsternal incision, excluding cases of emergency, active infection or with any history of cerebrovascular events. We retrospectively compared 45 patients undergoing C-RCP from January 1999 to April 2002 with 36 patients undergoing IPA-RCP from May 2002 to December 2006. Univariable and multivariable analysis were performed to examine statistically about the incidence of neurological morbidity, that is, delayed awakening, stroke and postoperative delirium.

Results (NS: not significant)

	C-RCP	IPA-RC`	p value
30 day mortality	2.22%	2.78%	NS
Time length needed to awake	7.1+/−4.9	3.8+/−2.9	0.013
Postoperative ventilatory support time	61+/−146	33+/−59	NS
Operative dosage of fentanyl	24.0+/−10.7	16.2+/−7.5	0.0009
Operative dosage of morphine	17.3+/−11.7	1.3+/−5.0	<0.0001
Operation time	508+/−221	457+/−146	NS
Cardiopulmonary bypass time	262+/−109	243+/−73	NS
Myocardial ischemia time	143+/−68	145+/−22	NS
RCP time	53+/−20	59+/−16	NS
Stroke	4.4%	2.9%	NS
Paraplegia	4.4%	2.9%	NS
Postoperative delirium	31.1%	8.3%	0.02

S. Takamoto, K. Nawata, T. Morota, K. Kitahori, and M. Kawata
The Department of Cardiothoracic Surgery, The University of Tokyo Hospital, Tokyo, Japan

Clinical outcomes of C group and IPA group were similar in mortality and operative data. As for postoperative delirium, univariable analysis revealed conventional RCP group, concomitant CABG, concomitant valve surgery and intraopertive body weight gain were correlated. Multivariable analysis for delirium showed conventional RCP group and concomitant CABG as risk factors, but not for the dosages of fentanyl and morphine. In conclusion, Conventional RCP and IPA-RCP demonstrated comparable postoperative outcomes after aortic arch repair via median sternotomy. IPA-RCP was suggested to contribute to the low frequency of delirium after aortic arch repair.

Modified Arch First Technique for Total Arch Replacement using Hypothermic Circulatory Arrest and Retrograde Cerebral Perfusion

Yuichi Ueda

Summary Patients and methods: From 1998 to 2007, there were 90 consecutive patients who underwent the modified arch first technique for total arch replacement using hypothermic circulatory arrest (HCA) and retrograde cerebral perfusion (RCP). There were 63 true aneurysms, and 13 chronic and 11 acute Stanford type A dissections. Sixteen cases were operated on as emergencies.

Results: The mean operation time was approximately 6.5 hr. The mean cardiopulmonary bypass time exceeded 3.5 hr as a result of applying HCA, with an average lowest esophageal temperature of 19.2°C. The mean HCA time with RCP was 31.2 ± 8.6 min. However, the lower body ischemic time was 80 min because of double segment distal anastomoses were performed. The cardiac ischemic time was nearly 2 hr. There were 4 hospital deaths. Nine patients (10%) suffered from stroke. Reversible ischemic neurological deficit was complicated during the operation in six cases (7%).

Conclusions: A recently refined arch first technique under HCA and RCP is still developing, but some refinements definitely contribute to better clinical outcomes. According to current information, the use of RCP for cerebral protection during HCA is safe when flow rates and central venous pressures are maintained at relatively low levels. (190 words)

Keywords Aortic surgery · Brain protection · Hypothermic circulatory arrest · Retrograde cerebral perfusion

---

Y. Ueda (✉)
Professor and Chairman
Division of Cardiac Surgery, Department of Surgery
Nagoya University Graduate School of Medicine
65 Tsurumai-cho, Showa-ku, Nagoya, Japan 466-8550
e-mail: yueda@med.nagoya-u.ac.jp

Introduction

Total arch replacement remains a challenging procedure in aortic surgery, although surgical results are improving following recent technical improvements [1]. We have introduced total arch replacement by reconstructing the arch and arch vessels with a four-branched graft under deep hypothermic circulatory arrest (HCA) with retrograde cerebral perfusion (RCP) through a median sternotomy [2,3]. Retrograde cerebral perfusion provides a better operative field without complicated cannulae into the arch vessels, although there are time limitations on safe HCA. The safe interval has been reported to be less than 60 min [4–6]. A shorter period of circulatory arrest should give better brain protection and faster neurological recovery after surgery. Therefore, to reduce the HCA with RCP time, we have adopted a modified arch first technique [7] through median sternotomy [8] since 1998, instead of the conventional distal anastomosis first technique. We evaluate surgical results of total arch replacement with the modified arch first technique.

Patients and Methods

From 1998 to 2007, there were 90 consecutive patients who underwent the modified arch first technique for total arch replacement. Of these, 59 were male and 31 female, with an average age of 67±8.0 years. There were 63 true aneurysms, and 13 chronic and 11 acute Stanford type A dissections. Sixteen cases were operated on as emergencies [Table 1].

Precise operative technique has been published previously [8]. Outline of the procedure was summarized as followed. After a median sternotomy and careful inspection of the ascending aorta with epi-aortic echo, cardiopulmonary bypass was applied with bicaval drainage and the ascending aortic return. The aortic arch was touched as little as possible to minimize the dislodgement of debris prior to initiation of circulatory arrest. Perfusion was discontinued once the esophageal temperature fell below 21°C by core cooling. Bi-spectral EEG analysis with spectral

Table 1 Patients characteristics

	n = 90
Age y.o. (m±SD)	67±8.0
Gender male/female	59/31
Pathology of Aneurysm	
Non-dissection (rupture)	63(2)
Dissection (acute)	24(11)
PAU	2
other	1
Emergency	16

PAU: Penetrating aortic ulcer

edge frequency and power of EEG using BIS monitor (A-1050, Aspect Medical Systems Inc., U.S.A.) showed a nearly flat level of EEG activity, circulatory arrest should be established. Cold blood cardioplegia was given. The arch vessels were transected at their origin, and each vessel was reconstructed with a four branched arch graft (Hemashield, Boston Science, Co. U.S.A. or Gelwaeve, Vascutek, Co. U.K.) with a 4–0 polypropylene running suture in the following sequence: left subclavian artery, left carotid artery, and brachiocephalic artery. Retrograde cerebral perfusion was applied via the superior vena cava (SVC) cannula snared with an umbilical tape after reconstructing the left subclavian artery. The SVC pressure was maintained at approximately 10–15 mmHg with 250–400 ml/min of flow rate by clamping the inferior vena cava cannula. The blood temperature was held at around 16°C. After anastomoses of the arch vessels, the flow rate of RCP was increased to 500–700 ml min to complete de-airing and flush debris; the RCP was then discontinued and antegrade cerebral perfusion was resumed through the four branched arch graft, with clamping at both ends of the main graft. The perfusion flow was maintained at 15 ml/kg/min so that the left radial artery pressure was above 30–40 mmHg (Fig. 1 a,b,c).

Distal anastomosis was performed using an elephant trunk technique. Distal perfusion to the lower body commenced with a Foley catheter inserted into the elephant trunk graft. The elephant trunk graft and the arch graft were anastomosed and then total cardiopulmonary bypass was resumed through the branched arch graft and the patient was rewarmed fully. The ascending aorta was then transected and proximal anastomosis between the arch graft and the aortic root was completed (Fig.1 d,e,f). Cardiopulmoary bypass was weaned off as usual fashion.

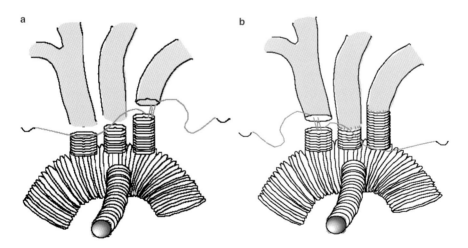

Fig. 1a and b The arch vessels were transected at their origin, and each vessel was reconstructed with a four branched arch with a 4–0 polypropylene running suture in the following sequence: left subclavian artery, left carotid artery, and brachiocephalic artery. Retrograde cerebral perfusion was applied after reconstructing the left subclavian artery

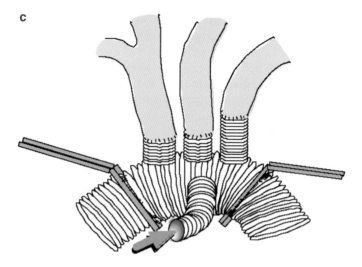

Fig. 1c Antegrade cerebral perfusion was resumed through the four branched arch graft with clamping at both ends of the main graft

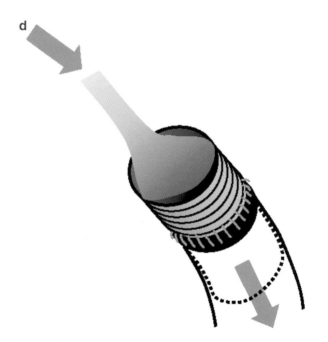

Fig. 1d Distal anastomosis was performed using an elephant trunk technique. Distal perfusion to the lower body commenced with a Foley catheter inserted into the elephant trunk graft

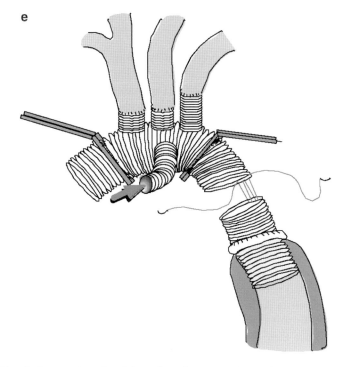

Fig. 1e The elephant trunk graft and the arch graft were anastomosed

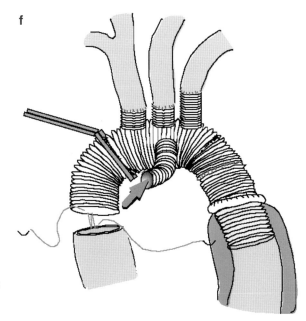

Fig. 1f The proximal anastomosis between the arch graft and the aortic root was completed

Results

The mean operation time was approximately 6.5 hr. The mean cardiopulmonary bypass time exceeded 3.5 hr as a result of applying HCA, with an average lowest esophageal temperature of 19.2°C. The mean HCA time with RCP was 31.2 ± 8.6 min. However, the lower body ischemic time was 80 min because of double segment distal anastomoses were performed. The cardiac ischemic time was nearly 2 hr, during which all of the aortic arch reconstruction procedures were performed. [Table 2]

There were 4 hospital deaths. Nine patients (10%) suffered from stroke, mainly minor focal embolic stroke. Reversible ischemic neurological deficit was complicated during the operation in six cases (7%). [Table 3]

Discussion

Retrograde cerebral perfusion was first used as a method to flush out accidental massive air embolism during cardiopulmonary bypass. We introduced this method as an adjunct to improve cerebral protection during HCA for the aortic arch surgery in 1989 [2]. Since then, RCP has been adopted with great enthusiasm. The most ardent proponents of RCP are convinced that RCP is effective in reducing embolic injury and in prolonging the permissible period of HCA. Many clinical reports have suggested that RCP in combination with HCA significantly decreases the rate of stroke and operative mortality associated with aortic arch operation [4–6, 9–13].

Table 2 Operative Data

Nasopharyngeal temperature (°C)	19.2 ± 1.1
CA time (min)	31.2 ± 8.6
\<RCP time (min)\>	\<14.5 ± 8.7\>
Lower body ischemia (min)	79.9 ± 28.5
Myocardial ischemia (min)	126.6 ± 41.6
Cardiopulmonary bypass (min)	226 ± 69
Operative time (min)	461 ± 179

CA: Circulatory arrest, RCP: Retrograde cerebral Perfusion

Table 3 Operative results

Hospital deaths	4 cases (4.4%)
Late deaths	8 cases (8.8%)
Complications	
renal failure	4 cases
re-exploration	10 cases
LOS	2 cases
Stroke	9 cases
TND	6 cases

TND: Transient neurological disturbance

In spite of clinical results have been improved after introduction of RCP, it is impossible to separate the effect of the learning curve from the effect of RCP that was usually introduced as surgeons became more proficient in the performance of the procedures.

Experimental investigations for effectiveness of RCP with animal model were also published [14,15]. Those experimental protocol were too long RCP time, such as 90 to 120 minutes and high RCP pressure to promote brain injury and edema. There exists much evidence that RCP per se seems to carry an increased risk of perfusion-induced cerebral injury, especially if high perfusion pressures are used. We always advocated the upper limits of the internal jugular vein pressure less than 20 mmHg. Even with unfavorable condition of HCA and RCP protocol in animal experimental models, those results of brain function with RCP were better than those of HCA without RCP [14,15]. It is clear that the details of RCP implementation are very critical to provide benefit without inducing damage from the cerebral edema.

The arch-first technique was introduced by Rokkas and Kouchoukos [7] in 1999 to minimize cerebral ischemic time and the technical difficulty of the intricate distal anastomosis. The rationale of this technique is to perform the brachiocephalic vessel connections first, and then to use selective antegrade cerebral perfusion through the completed graft while the distal anastomosis is being constructed. Kouchoukos and Masetti [16] reported superior clinical results to those with arch first technique with a branched graft that uses antegrade brain perfusion without the need for direct cannulation of the brachiocephalic arteries or a separate perfusion circuit, with only a brief period of circulatory arrest of the brain. We perform total arch replacement by reconstructing the arch vessels first with a four branched graft under HCA with RCP only through a median sternotomy [8]. We have always sought to improve surgical technique, especially cerebral protection which remains a major concern in aortic arch surgery. Hypothermic circulatory arrest with RCP is a simple technique. It can be performed without complicated perfusion circuits, and provides a better operative field for the graft anastomosis site with cervical vessels or the descending aorta [8]. We have proposed that RCP, with less than 20 mmHg pressure, should not exceed 60 min when sufficient flow is not present, because it is absolute non-physiological perfusion. We believe that a shorter period of RCP is better for cerebral protection and neurological recovery after surgery [4–6, 9–13]. Therefore, we adopted the arch first technique so as to shorten the period of HCA with RCP. This success shifts the goal from reducing surgical mortality and morbidity to improving the quality of life after the aortic arch surgery.

Conclusions

A recently refined arch first technique under HCA and RCP is still developing, however, some refinements definitely contribute to better clinical outcomes. According to current information, the use of RCP for cerebral protection during HCA is safe when flow rates and central venous pressures are maintained at relatively low levels.

References

1. Ueda Y, Osada H, Osugi H (2007) Japanese Association for Thoracic Surgery Committee of Science. Thoracic and cardiovascular surgery in Japan during 2005. Annual report by the Japanese Association for Thoracic Surgery. Gen Thorac Cardiovasc Surg 55:377–399
2. Ueda Y, Miki S, Kusuhara K, et al (1990) Surgical treatment of aneurysm or dissection involving the ascending aorta and aortic arch, utilizing circulatory arrest and retrograde cerebral perfusion. J Cardiovasc Surg (Torino) 31:553–558
3. Ueda Y, Miki S, Kusuhara K, et al (1992) Deep hypothermic systemic circulatory arrest and continuous retrograde cerebral perfusion for surgery of aortic arch aneurysm. Eur J Cardiothorac Surg 6: 36–41
4. Okita Y, Takamoto S, Ando M, et al (1998) Mortality and cerebral outcome in patients who underwent aortic arch operations using deep hypothermic circulatory arrest with retrograde cerebral perfusion: no relation of early death, stroke, and delirium to the duration of circulatory arrest. J Thorac Cardiovasc Surg 115:129–138
5. Ueda Y, Okita Y, Aomi S, et al (1999) Retrograde cerebral perfusion for aortic arch surgery: analysis of risk factors. Ann Thorac Surg 67:1879–1882
6. Bavaria JE, Pochettino A (1997) Retrograde cerebral perfusion (RCP) in aortic arch surgery: efficacy and possible mechanisms of brain protection. Semin Thorac Cardiovasc Surg 9:222–32
7. Rokkas CK, Kouchoukos NT (1999) Single-stage extensive replacement of the thoracic aorta: the arch-first technique. J Thorac Cardiovasc Surg 117:99–105
8. Sasaki M, Usui A, Yoshikawa M, et al (2005) Arch-first technique performed under hypothermic circulatory arrest with retrograde cerebral perfusion improves neurological outcomes for total arch replacement. Eur J Cardiothorac Surg 27:821–5
9. Coselli JS, Büket S, Djukanovic B (1995) Aortic Arch Operation: Current Treatment and Results. Ann Thorac Surg 59:19–27
10. Pagano D, Carey JA, Patel RL, et al (1995) Retrograde cerebral perfusion: clinical experience in emergency and elective aortic operations. Ann Thorac Surg 59:393–397
11. Deeb GM, Jenkins E, Bolling SF, et al (1995) Retrograde cerebral perfusion during hypothermic circulatory arrest reduces neurologic morbidity. J Thorac Cardiovasc Surg 109:259–268
12. Lytle BW, McCarthy PM, Meaney KM, et al (1995) Systemic hypothermia and circulatory arrest combined with arterial perfusion of the superior vena cava. Effective intraoperative cerebral protection. J Thorac Cardiovasc Surg 109:738–743
13. Safi HJ, Letsou GV, Iliopoulos DC, et al (1997) Impact of retrograde cerebral perfusion on ascending aortic and arch aneurysm repair. Ann Thorac Surg 63:1601–1607
14. Sakurada T, Kazui T, Tanaka H, et al (1996) Comparative experimental study of cerebral protection during aortic arch reconstruction. Ann Thorac Surg 61:1348–1354
15. Juvonen T, Zhang N, Wolfe D, et al (1998) Retrograde cerebral perfusion enhances cerebral protection during prolonged hypothermic circulatory arrest: a study in a chronic porcine model. Ann Thorac Surg 66:38–50
16. Kouchoukos NT, Masetti P (2004) Total aortic arch replacement with a branched graft and limited circulatory arrest of the brain. J Thorac Cardiovasc Surg 128:233–7

Symposium 3
State of Arts: Treatment for Thoracoabdominal and Abdominal Aorta

Endovascular Repair for Thoracoabdominal Aortic Aneurysms

Toru Kuratani, Yukitoshi Shirakawa, Kazuo Shimamura,
Mugiho Takeuchi, Goro Matsumiya, and Yoshiki Sawa

Thoracoabdominal aortic aneurysms (TAAA) are extremely burdensome to treat, due to their surgical complexity. In particular, postoperative spinal paraplegia poses severe complications that significantly lower patient QOL. Therefore, we focused on stent grafting, which is associated with a low incidence of postoperative paraplegia we devised a surgical procedure consisting of extended endovascular aortic repair (EVAR) and an abdominal visceral bypass. This presentation reports on the positive results attained from this procedure. 542 EVARs were conducted between January 1997 and September 2007. Among these, we selected 64 cases of TAAA, of which 38 were Crawford type I, 11 were Crawford type II, and 15 were Crawford type III. The average age of patients was 74.6 years. Preoperative complications included 8 cases of cerebrovascular damage, 7 cases of CAD, 8 cases of COPD. For spinal cord protection, Cerebrospinal fluid drainage and dosage of naloxone was initiated during the operation. Of Crawford I patients, we inserted stent grafts above the celiac artery in 25 of these cases, and above SMA with sacrifice of the celiac artery in 13 cases. For Crawford II, III patients, we performed bypassing from the aortic bifurcation to abdominal visceral arteries before deploying the stent graft. Operative time averaged 86 minutes for EVAR only and 328 minutes with bypass. There was no death and only a single case of graft occlusion. There were no cases of endoleak, and 47 cases shrinked aneurysms. Furthermore, not a single patient exhibited paraplegia and delayed paraplegia. In conclusion, we obtained satisfying results by EVAR for TAAA. Even though sufficient follow-up is needed for visceral bypasses, the procedure might be one of the standard surgeries for thoracoabdominal aortic aneurysms.

T. Kuratani, Y. Shirakawa, K. Shimamura, M. Takeuchi, G. Matsumiya, and Y. Sawa
Department of Cardiovascular Surgery, Osaka University, Osaka Japan

Multicenter Clinical trial of Zenith AAA Endovascular Graft for Abdominal Aortic Aneurysm in Japan

Kimihiko Kichikawa, Shoji Sakaguchi, Wataru Higashiura, and Hideo Uchida

Endovascular aneurysm repair (EVAR) has been widely adopted as a minimally invasive therapy for abdominal aortic aneurysm (AAA), however, evaluation of EVAR for AAA in Asian people have been poorly studied. And there are some reports about the anatomical differences of aorto-iliac region between western and Asian people.

We analyzed the multicenter data that was prospectively collected in four institutes in Japan to assess the safety and effectiveness of the Zenith stent graft (Zenith) for AAA. Ninety-seven patients (93 men, mean age 74 years, range 54–86) have undergone EVAR using Zenith. Aneurysm diameter ranged from 40 to 76 mm with a mean of 51 mm. Patients were evaluated for change in aneurysm size, endoleak, graft migration, conversion, rupture, and device integrity.

In all 97 patients, Zenith stent grafts were placed correctly at the target site and technical success rate is 100%. Procedural success rate is 99% (95/96) and 1 patient had Type I endoleak. There was no perioperative death in the series. The incidence of endoleak was 12% (Type II; 10, Type I; 1) at 6 month and 10.9% (Type II; 9, Type I; 1) at 1 year. Mean major axis of aneurysm changed from 51.1 ± 8.4 mm to 44.7 ± 10.3 mm after 1 year significantly. The size of AAA decreased or remained unchanged in 97.8%. No downward migration of stent graft was recorded. Iliac artery dissection or stenosis in 3 patients were successfully treated with Wallstent.

On the basis of follow-up results in this trial, Zenith appears to be safe and effective in treating AAA in Japan.

K. Kichikawa, S. Sakaguchi, W. Higashiura, and H. Uchida
Department of Radiology, Nara Medical University

Panel Discussion 1
Advanced Understanding and Consensus on IMH/PAU

Advanced Understanding and Consensus on IMH/PAU

Case Presentation

Sachio Kuribayashi

With recent progress of imaging techniques such as CT, echo and MRI, the condition termed as intramural hematoma (IMH) has been recognized. In this pathological condition, aortic media is dissected by the hematoma as the result of bleeding from vasa vasorum of the aortic wall, but the intima is intact without any tear. The term of IMH tends to be used too easy without precise interpretation of the imaging findings. There might be some confusion between IMH and thrombosed type dissection with intimal tear which is not well recognized on images. IMH could disappear spontaneously with medical treatment but it is now recognized as a variant of aortic dissection, because it could progress to overt dissection or aortic aneurysm.

The concept of penetrating atherosclerotic ulcer (PAU) was first proposed by Stanson, et al. in 1986. Pathological feature is characterized by ulceration in the aortic atheroma, which deepens through the elastic lamina into the media. This could cause medial hematoma, adventitial false aneurysm, and transmural rupture. Clinically, it is frequently seen in older patients over 65 years old with severe atherosclerosis of the aorta. The development of aortic dissection related to PAU is controversial, and ulcer-like projection (ULP) in thrombosed type dissection is sometimes confused with PAU on CT and angiography.

In this panel discussion, several cases will be presented for discussion and advanced understanding of IMH and PAU.

S. Kuribayashi (✉)
Professor and Chairman of Radiology, Keio University School of Medicine

Recent Advances in Imaging Aortic Diseases

David M. Williams

Advances in imaging aortic diseases can be presented from several perspectives: technical developments which open new windows into diagnosing and monitoring treatment of aortic disease, and recent anatomical and pathophysiological insights into aortic disease made possible by systematic imaging-pathological correlation of diseased aorta. This talk will focus on a review of recent advances in multi-detector helical CT, MRI, and molecular imaging as they bear on aortic disease, principally aortitis and atherosclerosis, as well as on recent work showing how CT findings corroborate and explain TEE observations in intramural hemorrhage involving the aorta.

D.M. Williams (✉)
Professor of Radiology, University of Michigan Medical School, Ann Arbor, MI

Intramural Hematoma and Penetrating Ulcer

VIII International Symposium on Advances in Understanding Aortic Diseases Tokyo, 2007

Thoralf M. Sundt, III

Sundt PAU and IMH Summary Intramural hematoma and penetrating ulcer represent the so-called variant forms of aortic dissection which complete the triad accountable for the vast majority of acute aortic syndromes. Although they may also occur in chronic forms, their management is most often discussed in the context of the acute presentation. Penetrating ulcers are uncommon and most frequently occur in the elderly with advanced occlusive atherosclerotic disease. They most often present in the descending thoracic aorta and are accompanied by at least a local intramural hemorrhage. There continues to be controversy over their natural history. The most recent series from the Mayo Clinic suggests that the majority may be managed in the acute setting nonoperatively with aggressive blood pressure control. Nonetheless, they run the risk of late evolution to saccular pseudoaneurysm or dissection. Likewise, intramural hematomas most often occur in the descending thoracic aorta and can most often be treated nonoperatively. They too run the risk of progression to more extensive disease. When either of these entities involve the ascending aorta, surgical intervention is the conventional approach. The role of endovascular stent grafting for either of these conditions remains in evolution and is dependent on a more complete understanding of their natural history.

Introduction

Advances in imaging technologies have increased our awareness of entities previously identified only surgically and pathologically. These entities include penetrating aortic ulcer (PAU) and intramural hematoma (IMH). With this shift

---

T.M. Sundt, III (✉)
Professor of Surgery and Consultant, Vice-Chair Department of Surgery
Mayo Clinic, Rochester, MN, 507-255-7064
e-mail: Sundt.Thoralf@Mayo.edu

in diagnostic modality, there has also been a subtle definitional confusion as pathologic criteria give way to radiologic criteria.. This is more than a matter of mere semantics; underlying these definitions are presumptions regarding pathogenic mechanisms that were established on a histopathologic basis but persist even as our diagnostic criteria have shifted to radiologic ones. Accordingly, we are now in a time of great controversy over the natural history of these conditions. This is a particularly relevant issue as new therapeutic interventions are introduced, the appropriate application of which should be based on a thorough understanding of the results of nonoperative management. Furthermore, at the same time as definitions have shifted, these entities are being identified at earlier and earlier stages of their evolution adding another dimension to the complexity of these questions.

The principle focus of this essay is the two so-called variant forms of aortic dissection, penetrating aortic ulcer (PAU) and intramural hematoma (IMH).[1] It is important to recognize that while all three of these entities may in some form or fashion coexist, and indeed one may evolve to another, the commonality of a final pathway does not necessitate common pathogenesis. For example, it might be argued from a theoretical basis that intramural hematoma and acute dissection be primarily considered an abnormality of the media.[2] While intimal disruption to create an entry site (or some would argue an exit site) occurs, the intima itself is often remarkably smooth and normal-appearing grossly. Indeed it is a common observation that most patients with acute dissection are remarkably free of atherosclerotic disease, and some have argued that thoracic aortic aneurysmal disease is in general terms not an atherosclerotic process.[3, 4] In contrast, penetrating aortic ulcer occurs typically among somewhat older patient population with extensive atherosclerotic disease suggesting that it is a disease primarily of the intima.

This theoretical distinction is not to disassociate the entities. Clearly, IMH is an entity clearly closely related to both acute dissection and PAU. Histopathologically, IMH is remarkably similar to acute dissection with fragmentation of elastin fibers and disruption of the media. Indeed, radiologic distinction between the two is difficult if not epistemologically impossible, as it relies on demonstrating the absence of an intimal defect if one adheres to Kruckenberg's classic definition of IMH.[5] Furthermore, evolution from intramural hematoma to acute dissection under observation is well documented and while the majority view today is that acute dissection begins with an intimal tear leading to development of a dissection plane, others continue to argue cogently that the contrary mechanism is just as reasonable an explanation, with all acute dissections beginning as intramural hematoma with subsequent rupture into the lumen allowing entry of luminal blood into an already disrupted intima and progression of the dissection plane. In point of fact, there are no hard data either way and one view is just as tenable as the other.

With regard to PAU, most often there is at least localized IMH present with PAU in the acute setting.[6, 7] If extensive, such IMH may progress to frank acute dissection completing the connection among the three entities.[8] These observations have led us to argue that these conditions might be most usefully considered along a multi-dimensional set of axes rather than being considered as a simple one-dimensional spectrum of disease.

The entities PAU, IMH and acute dissection are often referred to as lying along a "spectrum" of disease, a term conjuring up an image of a linear relationship. We have previously argues that it is more useful to consider these entities within a two-dimensional plane considering intimal disease along one and medial disease along a second axis.[2] While these entities can certainly be related to one another as noted above, at a minimum this conceptualization reduces our definitions to frankly observable anatomic and pathologic phenomena. Intramural hematoma without involvement of the intima clearly lies in a separate location from acute dissection with intimal disruption, et cetera. Movement from one region of the plane to another may be observed objectively but if not presumed. Given the confusion that exists surrounding the behavior of these entities, and the clinically apparent differences in outcome given location, we have expanded this concept further to now consider location in the aorta along a third axis (Fig. 1).

A final element to consider, which is no less critical to the issue of therapeutic management, is that of time which might be considered as the fourth dimension. While these three entities are commonly discussed in the context of acute aortic syndrome[9], all may be identified in chronic forms. One has every reason to believe that these entities may behave quite differently as chronic conditions rather than as acute ones. For example, it is commonly observed that the likelihood of progression to acute pericardial tamponade is far less for an incidentally identified chronic Type A dissection than for an acute one. Accordingly, it is common clinical practice to operate emergently on the acute form while the chronic form is scheduled on a semi-elective basis. Is it not equally logical that chronic and acute

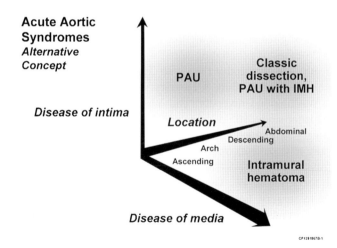

Fig. 1 The entities acute dissection, imtramural hematoma and penetrating aortic ulcer may be considered as overlapping manifestations of a spectrum of disease, however the spectrum should be considered along three physical axes as shown, as well as a temporal axis (acute vs. chronic). Such a construct reflects observable phenomena and not presumed pathogenetic mechanisms. We suggest that defining our terms according to such a construct will best facilitate accurate discovery of the behavior of these entities

intramural hematomas and penetrating ulcers may similarly behave differently and accordingly their appropriate management may differ? At the very least, these distinctions should be made within the literature as we struggle to define the natural history of these conditions and define appropriate therapeutic modalities. A framework such as this would confine us to objectively observable characteristics without presumptions concerning pathogenesis.

Penetrating Aortic Ulcer

It is commonly held that Shumacker first described penetrating aortic ulcer, however all would agree that the modern pathologic and radiologic description of this entity as well as recommendations for surgical management were most clearly described by Stanson in 1986.[6] He and his colleagues recognized an entity appearing on aortography much as a gastric ulcer appears on upper GI barium studies. They observed that this entity had an aggressive and malignant behavior with high mortality mandating surgical therapy, and importantly also noted that it frequently occurred in the distal thoracic aorta emphasizing the importance of including this portion of the thoracic aorta in the surgical repair. Within a short time, however, an alternate view of the natural history of this condition was expressed by Hussain and colleagues[10]. Their perspective, which was supported by observations reported by Kazerooni and colleagues[11] demonstrated a less aggressive condition which could often be managed nonoperatively initiating a controversy that continues to this day.

The more recent information comes from the highly respected investigators at Yale University's center for thoracic aortic diseases. Their 2002 publication supported Stanson's original argument arguing for surgical therapy in almost all cases. Among their 26 cases of penetrating aortic ulcer, they observed a greater risk of rupture or death with this entity than with Type B dissection.[12] Indeed, in their series, 40% experienced rupture. A contrary view was supported by our modest experience at Washington University[13] and subsequently a larger series at the Mayo Clinic[7]. In the latter study, 105 patients with PAU were identified by retrospective review of primary radiographic images by Stanson. Only 9% of these experienced rupture. Twenty-nine patients underwent surgical intervention, the majority in the earlier experience. The surgical mortality was quite high at 21% while that for nonoperative therapy was 4%. There is obvious selection bias here as the sickest patients went to surgery, however the data do demonstrate that in a significant percentage of cases medical management is possible.

Perhaps the most ready explanation for this difference in observed behavior is simply one of referral bias and the threshold of detection. It would be no surprise that the mortality rate was high among the patients identified by Stanson, as one would expect the earliest notice of a condition to be made among those with the most extreme symptomotology. Indeed such an observation would have been largely dependent upon surgical and autopsy studies eliminating from view any cases of lesser extent that might have been managed less aggressively. With growing awareness of the entity and its ante-mortem radiologic hallmarks, it is likely that the diagnosis was made subsequently at an earlier and earlier stage. This phenomenon is universal, as earlier radiologic diagnoses of all manner of medical entities are changing our view of their natural history and, accordingly, management. The same is likely operative in the Yale vs. Mayo controversy. At Yale, fully one-third of their patients presented with rupture, making it no surprise that a high risk of rupture came out of the analysis, or that two-thirds underwent surgical intervention. Furthermore, in almost half of the Yale patients the penetrating aortic ulcer was identified in the ascending segment of the aorta, a location associated with worse behavior. In the Mayo series, only 2% were type A.

The clinical impact of this debate over natural history is made more relevant today with the advent of endovascular stent grafting. The lesion itself would appear irresistible for placement of the stent graft, however, very frequently it resides in the context of advanced atherosclerotic disease with stenotic and atheromatous access vessels in elderly patients, the patients often at the greatest risk of cerebrovascular accident with extensive arch disease and frequently prior stroke. Results of stent grafting for penetrating ulcers have been reported by Demers and colleagues at Stanford with primary success in 92% of the 26 patients including six with ruptured penetrating ulcers.[14] Unfortunately, freedom from treatment failure was only 65% at five years. Admittedly, these were first generation devices but emphasize the generally poor condition of the patients undergoing these procedures. More recently a relatively large study from Essen similarly reported success in 21 of 22 patients with only one perioperative death.[15] This is far better than the 21% surgical mortality in the Mayo series. There was, however, a 5% incidence of stroke. At 27 months of follow-up, there was only one late re-intervention. This calls into question the advisability of treating the symptomatic patients. Piffaretti reported treatment of 11 penetrating ulcers but had major complications at five including one transient ischemic attack and four episodes of acute renal failure.[16] Indeed, a review of the literature shows mortality rates varying from 0–12% and morbidity from 0–45%.

Accordingly, it is our recommendation and our practice at Mayo Clinic to treat patients with PAU expectantly. Asymptomatic patients with penetrating ulcers are monitored for evidence of development of pseudoaneurysm, intramural hematoma or aneurysmal dilatation. Should such occur, we proceed to endovascular therapy. For symptomatic patients, aggressive blood pressure control is the first intervention. If such ulcers become asymptomatic, and the vast majority do, they are treated as chronic asymptomatic patients noted above. If, however, the ulcer progresses or pain persists, they are treated endovascularly. It is also important to recognize that we make a marked distinction between those penetrating ulcers located in the ascending aorta versus those in the descending aorta. There are data to support the notion that Type A PAU progress just as is the case for Type A IMH and Type A acute dissection. We, therefore, treat the penetrating ulcers involving the ascending aorta operatively under semi-elective conditions. It should also be noted that not all luminal irregularities are PAU. The radiologic diagnosis of PAU depends upon making the distinction from thoracic aortic thrombus with irregularity of the surface.

Intramural Hematoma

Like PAU, controversy surrounds IMH. Classically defined by Krukenberg in 1920 on the basis of pathologic analysis as "a dissection without intramural tear"[5] the diagnosis now dependent upon radiologic criteria. As this shift has occurred, insistence on an intact intima has wavered, perhaps in part thanks to recognition that PAU is often accompanied by hemorrhage into the surrounding aortic wall.[6] Hence, while purists focus on radiologic test resolution to rule out intimal defect, others confound the issue by creating new terms such "intramural hematoma with giant ulcer." Although one can appreciate the origin of such a term, the mere use of the terms violates the very definition of IMH as first defined by Krukenberg! Others would argue that, since the distinction between intramural hematoma and acute dissection is imperfect, alternative terms such as "noncommunicating dissection" should be utilized. Frankly we are of the view that such a term may be quite useful given the apparent similarity of clinical behavior between IMH and acute dissection with thrombosed false lumen.

In most series, the majority of intramural hematomas involve the descending thoracic aorta. They have generally been thought to represent 5–10% of cases of acute aortic syndrome.[17–22] It is curious, however, that more recent reports from the Far East place the incidence much higher – in some cases as high as 30–40% of acute aortic syndromes appear to be IMH.[23–25] Some have suggested that IMH in the east represents a different disease, although the potential impact of differences in detection rates must be entertained.

It is generally held that intramural hematomas, at least those with the descending thoracic aorta, may be treated nonoperatively. A number of studies have documented better behavior of IMH as compared with acute dissection with malperfusion, aortic regurgitation, and stroke in IMH distinctly uncommon.[12, 17, 26–28] Given the remarkably low mortality rate associated with medical treatment of uncomplicated Type B dissection it is easy to accept this notion. In Estrera's recent study, the in-hospital mortality rate for uncomplicated type B dissection – which represented 53% of all type B dissections in their experience - was only 1.2%.[29] The acute behavior is likely in part dictated by flow dynamics which are of necessity similar to those of acute dissection with thrombosis of the false lumen.[30] Curiously the plane of dissection in IMH is said by some to be closer to the adventitia than that for dissection, an observation that is disconsonant with this clinical observation.[31, 32] Nonetheless, the overall outcome is generally felt better than acute dissection with Kaji reporting an in-hospital mortality rate of 0% and complete resolution in 50–70% of cases.[33] Although acute behavior in general is superior with intramural hematoma, this is not to trivialize the risk as IMH may progress rapidly to acute dissection or rupture.[26] Elefteriades has emphasized the importance of careful follow-up.[12]

What is the behavior of IMH in the chronic phase? Reported rates of progression over time to aneurysm may be in the range of 30–40%.[28, 34, 35] Conversely complete resolution of the hematoma has been observed in as many as half of patients within 6 months.[36, 37] Predictors of progression include presence of a penetrating ulcer[33] while predictors of resolution include younger age[33,37], diameter less than 4–4.5 cm[17,37,38] and hematoma thickness less than 1 cm[17,38]. It is important to note that Sueyoshi and colleagues suggested a biphasic modality in the behavior of patients with intramural hematoma including shrinkage in the first year but slow growth thereafter.[38] This emphasizes the importance of long-term monitoring. As compared with type B dissection, survival is superior for IMH at 1 year (100% vs 83%), two years, (97% vs 79%), and 5 years (97% vs 79%).[33] It must also be noted that pharmacologic therapy has been shown to impact late survival, with a beneficial impact of beta blockers clear.[28]

This leaves significant question as to the role of endovascular therapy for intramural hematoma. If half will resolve, can one justify acute treatment of the condition when the acute behavior is relatively benign? If one is treating for the sake of reducing the risk of late aneurysm formation, where would one best seat the endograft? The important serial CT scan study performed by Sueyoshi and colleagues demonstrated that while the region of the aorta destined to enlarge the most is that which is largest acutely, in as many as one-third it is not![39] What represents the proximal and distal landing zones? Would one cover the entire aorta with the attendant risks of paraplegia to treat a condition that may or may not progress? Furthermore, what is the appropriate diameter of such a graft if IMH is at risk for remodeling to an aneurysmal aorta as we all know it may? At this point in time, it seems meddlesome to intervene in the acute phase.

Greater controversy surrounds management of IMH involving the ascending aorta (not to mention the arch on which there are so little data that we will say nothing further about it). The first series of IMH reported very aggressive behavior of those involving the ascending aorta.[34,35] This view was supported by the majority of subsequent studies[8,12], including a multicenter European study[28] and recent meta-analysis.[20]

The counter-view arose out of experience in Japan and Korea, where success has been reported with a strategy of intensive nonoperative or expectant management of Type A IMH. In 1997 Sueyoshi reported the successful management of 8 patients with type A IMH treated nonoperatively with one death as compared with o deaths among 5 surgically treated patients.[40] The following year Moriyama reported on 18 patients with type A IMH, 6 of whom were treated surgically with one death, and 12 of whom were treated medically with no mortality.[41] Medical management of another 11 patients with three deaths was reported by Shimizu in 2000[25], and the largest series that of Song and colleagues from Korea in which 36 of 41 patients presenting with type A IMH were treated nonoperatively with only three deaths.[36] Kaji has reported only 2 deaths among 30 patients so treated.[27] Given these favorable experiences, these investigators have called for expectant therapy as a routine approach to type A IMH. Predictors of successful nonoperative management include diamtere less than 50 mm[27] and thickness less than 11–12 mm[42,43]

It is important in the context of this discussion to examine closely the treatment protocol, including indications for proceeding to surgery, as well as the long-term outcome of this approach. First, the treatment algorithm entails close observation in hospital for as much as one month, with bed rest for one to two weeks and frequent imaging studies throughout the hospitalization to monitor carefully for progression of the IMH.[42] Candidates for such an approach, according to these investigators, include all hemodynamically stable patients without evidence of tamponade. Indications to proceed with emergent surgical repair include tamponade and "impending rupture" as well as frank rupture. It should also be noted that a significant percentage of patients do, ultimately, end up in the operating room. In Kaji's series, 43% had surgery during their hospitalization and 60% eventually progressed,[27] as did 50% of those treated in Moizumi's series.[42] A significant number of late IMH-related deaths occurred in the latter series as well. There may be a cost in terms of operative risk as well, with this approach of necessity bringing patients to surgery under urgent or emergent circumstances rather than semi-electively. In Song's series the operative mortality rate was fully 20%[44], much higher than that reported by others in the 5% range.[31, 41]

How can we resolve this apparent paradox? What is the explanation for this apparent difference in behavior of Type A intramural hematoma in the East and West? Some have argued an "Asian factor"[45] with some sort of racial or epidemiologic difference in the condition itself, perhaps related to incidence of hypertension or salt-intake. Data to support this notion, however, are lacking as is a well-defined or proposed mechanism. A second possibility is the difference in the diagnostic threshold analogous to our explanation for differences in opinion regarding the behavior of penetrating ulcer. Support for this explanation derives from the higher proportion of IMH among acute aortic syndromes among patients in Far East series noted above. If, indeed, the significant number of IMH has progressed to acute dissection or, indeed, all acute dissections begin as IMH, it could well be that in the Far East, where a higher incidence of IMH is identified, the condition is being captured earlier in its evolution. Further support for this argument may be marshaled by simple inspection of the diameter of the aorta identified in these Asian series which is frequently smaller than that commonly observed in clinical practice in the US.

Finally, it is possible that there is simply no difference at all in the natural history but rather a difference in threshold for tolerating risk of nonoperative therapy and acceptance of monitoring a patient as they progress during hospitalization and observation. A critical element in the expectant approach is prolonged hospitalization with frequent imaging studies and a willingness to operate emergently. Most Western authors and, indeed a significant number of Japanese authors as well, would argue that this approach invites potential disaster as one substitutes an urgent but not emergent surgical repair for an emergent repair under shock conditions in a subset. In Western series of repair of acute dissection, the presence of hemodynamic collapse has been demonstrated to be a profound risk factor for operative death.[46]

The balance of risks and benefits for these two approaches depends critically upon the operative risk in any given hospital for the elective and emergent procedures. If the risk for the elective procedure is high, then certainly the balance tilts in favor of an expectant approach. If, on the other hand, the operative risk for an elective repair of an IMH among a hemodynamically stable patient is low, as is the case in a number of series, the argument for expectant therapy is less. It is our approach to operate on Type A intramural hematoma expediently upon diagnosis as the operative risk in our hands has proven to be low. In selected patient circumstances, however, we have elected to treat such patients nonoperatively. The data do suggest, however, that in selected patients such as the very elderly one may get away with it particularly if the size is small.

Conclusions

The "variant forms" of acute dissection PAU and IMH remain incompletely understood and vaguely defined even as new therapeutic strategies are being introduced. As investigators with interest in these entities the onus is upon us to define our terms clearly and detail our observations in such manner that the role of endovascular therapies may be fairly determined. The promiscuous application of these technologies without an adequate understanding of the behavior of these entities invites therapeutic misadventure and iatrogenic harm.

References

1. Svensson LG, Labib SB, Eisenhauer AC, et al (1999) Intimal tear without hematoma: an important variant of aortic dissection that can elude current imaging techniques. Circulation 99:1331–6
2. Sundt TM (2007) Intramural hematoma and penetrating atherosclerotic ulcer of the aorta. Ann Thorac Surg 83:S835–41; discussion S846–50
3. Agmon Y, Khandheria BK, Meissner I, et al (2003) Is aortic dilatation an atherosclerosis-related process? Clinical, laboratory, and transesophageal echocardiographic correlates of thoracic aortic dimensions in the population with implications for thoracic aortic aneurysm formation. J Am Coll Cardiol 42:1076–83
4. Achneck H, Modi B, Shaw C, et al (2005) Ascending thoracic aneurysms are associated with decreased systemic atherosclerosis. Chest 128:1580–6
5. Krukenberg E (1920) Beitrage zur Frage des Aneurysma dissecans. Beitr Pathol Anat Allg Pathol 67:329–51
6. Stanson AW, Kazmier FJ, Hollier LH, et al (1986) Penetrating atherosclerotic ulcers of the thoracic aorta: natural history and clinicopathologic correlations. Annals of Vascular Surgery 1:15–23
7. Cho KR, Stanson AW, Potter DD, et al (2004) Penetrating atherosclerotic ulcer of the descending thoracic aorta and arch. J Thorac Cardiovasc Surg 127:1393–9; discussion 1399–1401
8. Ganaha F, Miller DC, Sugimoto K, et al (2002) Prognosis of aortic intramural hematoma with and without penetrating atherosclerotic ulcer: a clinical and radiological analysis. Circulation 106:342–8
9. Vilacosta I, Roman JA (2001) Acute aortic syndrome. Heart 85:365–8
10. Hussain S, Glover JL, Bree R, Bendick PJ (1989) Penetrating atherosclerotic ulcers of the thoracic aorta. Journal of Vascular Surgery 9:710–7
11. Kazerooni EA, Bree RL, Williams DM (1992) Penetrating atherosclerotic ulcers of the descending thoracic aorta: evaluation with CT and distinction from aortic dissection. Radiology 183:759–65

12. Tittle SL, Lynch RJ, Cole PE, et al (2002) Midterm follow-up of penetrating ulcer and intramural hematoma of the aorta. Journal of Thoracic & Cardiovascular Surgery 123:1051–9
13. Absi TS, Sundt TM 3rd, Camillo C, et al (2004) Penetrating atherosclerotic ulcers of the descending thoracic aorta may be managed expectantly. Vascular 12:307–11
14. Demers P, Miller DC, Mitchell RS, et al (2004) Stent-graft repair of penetrating atherosclerotic ulcers in the descending thoracic aorta: mid-term results. Ann Thorac Surg 77:81–6
15. Eggebrecht H, Herold U, Schmermund A, et al (2006) Endovascular stent-graft treatment of penetrating aortic ulcer: results over a median follow-up of 27 months. Am Heart J 151:530–6
16. Piffaretti G, Tozzi M, Lomazzi C, et al (2007) Penetrating ulcers of the thoracic aorta: results from a single-centre experience. Am J Surg 193:443–7
17. Evangelista A, Mukherjee D, Mehta RH, et al (2005) Acute Intramural Hematoma of the Aorta. A Mystery in Evolution. Circulation 111:1063–70
18. Gore I (1952) Pathogenesis of dissecting aneurysm of the aorta. AMA Arch Pathol 53:142–53
19. Hirst AE Jr., Johns VJ Jr., Kime SW (1958) Dissecting aneurysm of the aorta: a review of 505 cases. Medicine (Baltimore) 37:217–279
20. Maraj R, Rerkpattanapipat P, Jacobs LE, et al (2000) Meta-analysis of 143 reported cases of aortic intramural hematoma. American Journal of Cardiology. 86:664–8
21. Sawhney NS, DeMaria AN, Blanchard DG (2001) Aortic intramural hematoma: an increasingly recognized and potentially fatal entity. Chest 120:1340–6
22. Vaccari G, Caciolli S, Calamai G, et al (2001) Intramural hematoma of the aorta: diagnosis and treatment. Eur J Cardiothorac Surg 19:170–3
23. Yamada T, Tada S, Harada J (1988) Aortic dissection without intimal rupture: diagnosis with MR imaging and CT. Radiology 168:347–52
24. Song JK, Kim HS, Kang DH, et al (2001) Different clinical features of aortic intramural hematoma versus dissection involving the ascending aorta. J Am Coll Cardiol 37:1604–10
25. Shimizu H, Yoshino H, Udagawa H, et al (2000) Prognosis of aortic intramural hemorrhage compared with classic aortic dissection. American Journal of Cardiology 85:792–5
26. Kaji S, Nishigami K, Akasaka T, et al (1999) Prediction of progression or regression of type A aortic intramural hematoma by computed tomography. Circulation 100:II281–6
27. Kaji S, Akasaka T, Horibata Y, et al (2002) Long-term prognosis of patients with type a aortic intramural hematoma. Circulation 106:I248–52
28. von Kodolitsch Y, Csosz SK, Koschyk DH, et al (2003) Intramural hematoma of the aorta: predictors of progression to dissection and rupture. Circulation 107:1158–63
29. Estrera AL, Miller CC, Goodrick J, et al (2007) Update on outcomes of acute type B aortic dissection. Ann Thorac Surg 83:S842–5; discussion S846–50
30. Juvonen T, Ergin MA, Galla JD, et al (1999) Risk factors for rupture of chronic type B dissections. J Thorac Cardiovasc Surg 117:776–86
31. Uchida K, Imoto K, Takahashi M, et al (2005) Pathologic characteristics and surgical indications of superacute type A intramural hematoma. Ann Thorac Surg 79:1518–21
32. Coady MA, Rizzo JA, Hammond GL, et al (1999) Surgical intervention criteria for thoracic aortic aneurysms: a study of growth rates and complications. Ann Thorac Surg 67:1922–6; discussion 1953–8
33. Kaji S, Akasaka T, Katayama M, et al (2003) Long-term prognosis of patients with type B aortic intramural hematoma. Circulation 108:9
34. Nienaber CA, von Kodolitsch Y, Petersen B, et al (1995) Intramural hemorrhage of the thoracic aorta. Diagnostic and therapeutic implications. Circulation 92:1465–72
35. Robbins RC, McManus RP, Mitchell RS, et al (1993) Management of patients with intramural hematoma of the thoracic aorta. Circulation 88:II1–II10.
36. Song JK, Kim HS, Song JM, et al (2002) Outcomes of medically treated patients with aortic intramural hematoma. Am J Med 113:181–7
37. Nishigami K, Tsuchiya T, Shono H, et al (2000) Disappearance of aortic intramural hematoma and its significance to the prognosis. Circulation 102:III243–7

38. Sueyoshi E, Imada T, Sakamoto I, et al (2002) Analysis of predictive factors for progression of type B aortic intramural hematoma with computed tomography. Journal of Vascular Surgery 35:1179–83
39. Sueyoshi E, Sakamoto I, Uetani M, Matsuoka Y (2006) CT analysis of the growth rate of aortic diameter affected by acute type B intramural hematoma. AJR Am J Roentgenol 186:S414–20
40. Sueyoshi E, Matsuoka Y, Sakamoto I, et al (1997) Fate of intramural hematoma of the aorta: CT evaluation. J Comput Assist Tomogr 21:931–8
41. Moriyama Y, Yotsumoto G, Kuriwaki K, et al (1998) Intramural hematoma of the thoracic aorta. Eur J Cardiothorac Surg 13:230–9
42. Moizumi Y, Komatsu T, Motoyoshi N, et al (2002) Management of patients with intramural hematoma involving the ascending aorta. J Thorac Cardiovasc Surg 124:918–24
43. Song JM, Kim HS, Song JK, et al (2003) Usefulness of the initial noninvasive imaging study to predict the adverse outcomes in the medical treatment of acute type A aortic intramural hematoma. Circulation 108:II324–8
44. Song JK, Kang SJ, Song JM, et al (2007) Factors associated with in-hospital mortality in patients with acute aortic syndrome involving the ascending aorta. Int J Cardiol 115:14–8
45. Mohr-Kahaly S (2001) Aortic intramural hematoma: from observation to therapeutic strategies. J Am Coll Cardiol 37:1611–3
46. Long SM, Tribble CG, Raymond DP, et al (2003) Preoperative shock determines outcome for acute type A aortic dissection. Ann Thorac Surg 75:520–4

Therapeutic Strategy of Acute Aortic Intramural Hematoma

Shuichiro Kaji

Summary The limited data on the natural history of intramural hematoma (IMH) suggest that it behaves very much like classic aortic dissection (AD) and should therefore be treated in a similar fashion. However, there is considerable controversy surrounding its prognosis and treatment. In order to investigate long-term clinical course in patients with IMH, we compared clinical data between type A IMH and AD patients and between type B IMH and AD patients. All type A IMH patients were treated initially with supportive medical therapy. All type B IMH or AD patients were treated with medical therapy. The actuarial survival rate in type A IMH patients was significantly higher than type A AD patients. The incidence of aortic regurgitation and stroke were significantly lower in IMH patients. On the other hand, the actuarial survival rate in type B IMH patients was significantly higher than type B AD patients. In summary, patients with IMH have different clinical features and better long-term prognosis than patients with AD. Considering mortality and morbidity for surgical repair, supportive medical treatment with frequent follow-up imaging studies can be a rational therapeutic strategy for type A IMH. Patients with type B IMH have favorable outcome with medical therapy.

Keywords Aortic intramural hematoma · aortic dissection · medical therapy · follow-up studies · prognosis

Introduction

Aortic intramural hematoma (IMH) was first described in 1920 as "dissection without intimal tear", and was considered a distinct entity at necropsy. [1] This is essentially a contained hemorrhage within the medial layer. Although the pathogenesis of IMH is still uncertain, rupture of the vasa vasorum is believed to be the initiating event. IMH

S. Kaji (✉)
Department of Cardiovascular Medicine, Kobe City Medical Center General Hospital
4-6, Minatojima-nakamachi, Chuo-ku, Kobe, Japan, 650-0046
e-mail: skaji@kcgh.gr.jp

is considered a precursor of classic dissection. [2] The presence of aortic IMH can weaken the medial layer and potentially increase the likelihood of a classic AD.

IMH is characterized by crescent aortic wall thickness without mobile flap, entry and flow communication. [3–5] In CT images, IMH is defined as segmental and crescent relatively low attenuation area without contrast enhancement. Transesophageal echocardiography also showed a crescent aortic wall thickening. [3] No intimal tear and no flow communication are prerequestic for the diagnosis of IMH. [6]

Similar to classic dissection, IMH may extend along the aorta, progress, regress, or reabsorb. [7–15] The limited data on the natural history of IMH suggest that it behaves very much like AD and should therefore be treated in a similar fashion. [4, 8, 10, 15] However, there is considerable controversy surrounding its prognosis and treatment. [9, 12, 14, 16–18] In this review, the clinical features, management, and prognosis will be discussed.

Clinical Features of IMH

The absence of intimal tear and continuous flow communication in patients with IMH may lead to different clinical features. Song et al. reported the clinical features of patients with IMH in comparison with AD. [13, 14] In this report, Patients with type A IMH were older, female dominant, more complicated with pericardial effusion and less complicated with aortic regurgitation than patients with aortic dissection. [14] Besides, patients with type B IMH were older than patients with AD. [13] We also compared the clinical features between patients with IMH and AD. Patients with type A IMH were significantly older than patients with AD. [9] In addition, the incidence of moderate to severe aortic regurgitation and stroke was lower in patients with IMH. On the other hand, in patients with type B aortic IMH, the incidence of serious complications including leg ischemia and renal failure was lower than patients with AD. [10]

Another important clinical features of aortic IMH is that hematoma may progress or regress with time. IMH evolves very dramatically in the short-term to regression, dissection or increase in hematoma size. [7] Figs. 1 and 2 shows the representative cases of complete resolution and progression of type A IMH.

Natural History of IMH

Different clinical features may have a different impact on clinical courses in patients with IMH. However, the natural history of acute IMH continues to be debated.

Nienaber et al. reported early clinical results of medical and surgical therapy in patients with IMH. [4] In this study, in patients with type A IMH, medically treated patients had worse prognosis than surgically treated patients. On the other hand, in patients with type B IMH, medically treated patients had similar short term prognosis with surgically treated patients. Thus, they concluded that early surgery

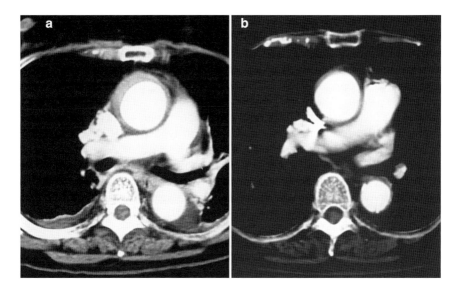

Fig. 1 One example of the regression of hematoma in a patient with type A IMH. Initial CT scan showed characteristic crescent wall thickening in both the ascending and descending aorta (**a**). Eight months later, follow-up study showed complete resolution of hematoma in both the ascending and descending aorta (**b**)

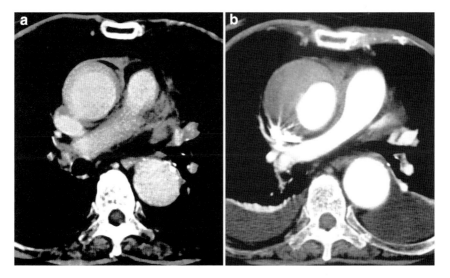

Fig. 2 One example of the progression of hematoma in a patient with type A IMH. Initial CT scan showed characteristic crescent wall thickening in both the ascending aorta (**a**). In this patient, IMH markedly increased with chest pain 7 days after the onset (**b**)

should be required in patients with type A IMH and patients with type B IMH can be controlled with medical therapy.

As for prognosis of patients with type B IMH, Song et al. reported the results of multi-center registry study. [18] In this study, almost 80% of patients with type B IMH showed disappearance of hematoma, whereas IMH progressed to AD in 20% of the patients. They also reported that 3 year survival rate was 87% in these patients. We investigated the long-term prognosis of patients with type B IMH. [10] We followed medically treated 53 patients with type B IMH. Mean follow-up period was almost 5 years. As a result, 77% of these patients showed regression of hematoma, whereas 23% of the patients showed progression. We compared the prognosis of these IMH patients with 57 type B AD patients. As a result, the actuarial survival rate in type B IMH patients at 5 years was significantly higher than type B AD patients (97% versus 79%, $p = 0.009$). Therefore, medically treated patients with type B IMH have good prognosis.

On the other hand, how to treat patients with type A IMH has been discussed for a long time. In terms of prognosis of patients with type A IMH, Song et al reported the results of medical therapy in patients with type A IMH. In this study, 67% of medically treated patients showed disappearance of hematoma. Three-year survival rate of medically treated patients was 78%. On the contrary, von Kodolitsch et al reported the different results of multi-center study in patients with type A IMH [15] In this study, medically treated patients have worse prognosis than surgically treated patients. In addition, the international registry of acute aortic dissection (IRAD) study reported the results of 23 patients with type A IMH. [8] In this study, in-hospital mortality of both medically and surgically treated patients were relatively high. Thus, they concluded that IMH is a highly lethal condition when it involves the ascending aorta and surgical therapy should be considered.

We investigated the long-term prognosis of patients with type A IMH. [9] We medically treated 30 patients with type A IMH and followed up for almost 5 years. We follow these patients initially with supportive medical therapy and close imaging follow-up. Patients who demonstrated the increased hematoma or progression to AD were referred for surgical repair and underwent urgent operation. As a result, in 30 patients, 13 patients developed classic aortic dissection or showed increased hematoma. These patients underwent graft replacement of the ascending aorta except for one patient who refused operation and died due to aortic rupture. Another 17 patients were treated medically. Finally, as shown in this slide, there were 2 early deaths and 1 late death. (Fig. 3) We compared the prognosis of these IMH patients with 101 type A AD patients. As a result, the actuarial survival rate in type A IMH patients at 5 years was significantly higher than type A AD patients (90% versus 62%, $p = 0.004$).

Table 1 shows the summary of medical therapy for patients with type A IMH. Mortality with medical therapy in patients with type A IMH varies from 0% to 80%. Especially, mortality rate is worse in European country than Japan and Korea. There is considerably controversy over the natural history of type A IMH.

The interesting results of meta-analysis about the international heterogeneity in diagnostic frequency and clinical outcomes of type A IMH were reported

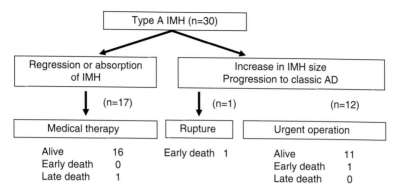

Fig. 3 Outcomes of patients with type A IMH who were treated initially with supportive medical therapy

Table 1 Summary of Medical Therapy for Patients With Type A IMH

Author	Year	Number of cases	Mean Age	Mortality with Medical Therapy	Resolution of hematoma
Mohr-Kahaly [3]	1994	3	72	2/3	NA
Nienaber [4]	1995	12	52	4/5	NA
Sueyoshi [21]	1997	13	70	1/8	4/8
Kaji [11]	1999	22	65	1/22	12/22
Shimiz [17]	2000	13	NA	3/11	NA
Hagan [22]	2000	17	NA	4/8	NA
Nishigami [12]	2000	8	72	1/8	2/8
Song [14]	2001	24	67	1/18	7/13
Sohn [23]	2001	13	NA	0/13	NA
Kaji [9]	2002	30	67	1/30	17/30
Song [18]	2002	41	65	3/41	24/36
Evangelista [7]	2003	12	NA	1/5	2/5
von Kodolitsch [15]	2003	38	NA	6/11	NA
Moizumi [16]	2004	41	67	3/30	NA
Evangelista [8]	2005	23	NA	3/9	NA

NA: not available

recently [19] In this study, frequency of aortic IMH was significantly higher in Japan and Korea than North America and European country. Medically treated patients were significantly more dominant in Japan and Korea and overall mortality rate was significantly lower in Japan and Korea. Why is there the difference of prognosis of patients with IMH involving the ascending aorta? It has been proposed that there might be a possible "Asian Factor". [1] We think that another possible reason for international heterogeneity might be the difference of availability of imaging modalities. Organization for Economic Cooperation and Development (OECD) reported in *OECD Health Data 2007* the numbers of CT scanners per million people in OECD countries. In this report, the numbers of CT scanners in Japan (92.6/million people) and Korea (32.2/million people) are over two times higher

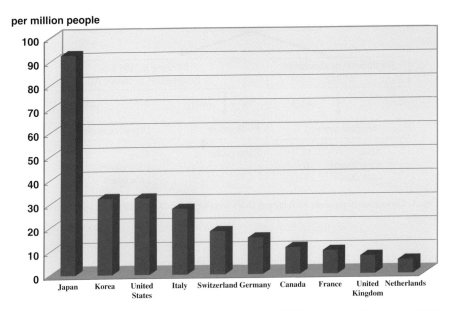

Fig. 4 The numbers of CT scanners per million people in OECD countries. (Data from *OECD Health Data 2007*: http://www.oecd.org)

than mean value of OECD countries (13.3/million people) (Fig. 4). High frequency of IMH in Japan and Korea may be due to high availability of CT scanners in emergency room, which may lead to possible early diagnosis of very mild IMH.

Risk Factors of Progression

To achieve better outcome in management of patients with type A IMH, it would be helpful to establish risk factors of the adverse outcomes. To clarify risk factors for progression in patients with type A IMH, we investigated clinical features and CT variables in initial images between patients with progression and regression. [11] As a result, there were no significant differences in clinical features. In CT variables, maximum aortic diameter and hematoma size in initial CT images were strong risk factors for progression. By multivariate analysis, the most significant predictor was the maximum aortic diameter. We found that maximum aortic diameter equal to or greater than 50 mm was the strongest risk factor for progression. Song et al reported similar results. [20] They investigated medically treated type A IMH patients and found that maximum aortic diameter equal to or greater than 48 mm and hematoma size equal to or greater than 11 mm were strong risk factors for progression. In this study, multivariate analysis identified hematoma size equal to or greater than 11 mm as the strongest risk factor.

Therapeutic Strategy

In summary, we would like to propose the therapeutic strategy for patients with IMH as follows; In type A IMH, surgical therapy should be recommended in complicated case with cardiac tamponade and/or aortic regurgitation. If patients are not complicated, medical therapy with frequent imaging follow-up can be a rational option. In these cases, surgery should be considered if hematoma may progress in size or progress to classic dissection. In addition, early surgery should be considered for high risk patients with aortic diameter equal to or greater than 50 mm and/or hematoma size equal to or greater than 11 mm. In type B IMH, patients should be treated medically if not complicated.

References

1. Mohr-Kahaly S (2001) Aortic intramural hematoma: from observation to therapeutic strategies. J Am Coll Cardiol 37: 1611–1613
2. Tsai TT, Nienaber CA, Eagle KA (2005) Acute aortic syndromes. Circulation 112: 3802–3813
3. Mohr-Kahaly S, Erbel R, Kearney P, et al (1994) Aortic intramural hemorrhage visualized by transesophageal echocardiography: findings and prognostic implications. J Am Coll Cardiol 23: 658–664
4. Nienaber CA, von Kodolitsch Y, Petersen B, et al (1995) Intramural hemorrhage of the thoracic aorta. Diagnostic and therapeutic implications. Circulation 92: 1465–1472
5. Robbins RC, McManus RP, Mitchell RS, et al (1993) Management of patients with intramural hematoma of the thoracic aorta. Circulation: II1–10
6. Kang DH, Song JK, Song MG, et al (1998) Clinical and echocardiographic outcomes of aortic intramural hemorrhage compared with acute aortic dissection. Am J Cardiol 81: 202–206
7. Evangelista A, Dominguez R, Sebastia C, et al (2003) Long-term follow-up of aortic intramural hematoma: predictors of outcome. Circulation 108: 583–589
8. Evangelista A, Mukherjee D, Mehta RH, et al (2005) Acute intramural hematoma of the aorta: a mystery in evolution. Circulation 111: 1063–1070
9. Kaji S, Akasaka T, Horibata Y, et al (2002) Long-term prognosis of patients with type A aortic intramural hematoma. Circulation 106: I248–252
10. Kaji S, Akasaka T, Katayama M, et al (2003) Long-term prognosis of patients with type B aortic intramural hematoma. Circulation 108 Suppl 1: II307–311
11. Kaji S, Nishigami K, Akasaka T, et al (1999) Prediction of progression or regression of type A aortic intramural hematoma by computed tomography. Circulation 100(Suppl II): II-281–II-286
12. Nishigami K, Tsuchiya T, Shono H, et al (2000) Disappearance of aortic intramural hematoma and its significance to the prognosis. Circulation 102: III243–247
13. Song JK, Kang DH, Lim TH, et al (1999) Different remodeling of descending thoracic aorta after acute event in aortic intramural hemorrhage versus aortic dissection. Am J Cardiol 83: 937–941
14. Song JK, Kim HS, Kang DH, et al (2001) Different clinical features of aortic intramural hematoma versus dissection involving the ascending aorta. J Am Coll Cardiol 37: 1604–1610
15. von Kodolitsch Y, Csosz SK, Koschyk DH, et al (2003) Intramural hematoma of the aorta: predictors of progression to dissection and rupture. Circulation 107: 1158–1163

16. Moizumi Y, Komatsu T, Motoyoshi N, et al (2004) Clinical features and long-term outcome of type A and type B intramural hematoma of the aorta. J Thorac Cardiovasc Surg 127: 421–427
17. Shimizu H, Yoshino H, Udagawa H, et al (2000) Prognosis of Aortic Intramural Hemorrhage Compared With Classic Aortic Dissection. Am J Cardiol 85: 792–795
18. Song JK, Kim HS, Song JM, et al (2002) Outcomes of medically treated patients with aortic intramural hematoma. Am J Med 113: 181–187
19. Pelzel JM, Braverman AC, Hirsch AT, et al (2007) International Heterogeneity in Diagnostic Frequency and Clinical Outcomes of Ascending Aortic Intramural Hematoma. J Am Soc Echocardiogr
20. Song JM, Kim HS, Song JK, et al (2003) Usefulness of the initial noninvasive imaging study to predict the adverse outcomes in the medical treatment of acute type A aortic intramural hematoma. Circulation 108 Suppl 1: II324–328
21. Sueyoshi E, Matsuoka Y, Sakamoto I, et al (1997) Fate of intramural hematoma of the aorta: CT evaluation. J Comput Assist Tomogr 21: 931–938
22. Hagan PG, Nienaber CA, Isselbacher EM, et al (2000) The International Registry of Acute Aortic Dissection (IRAD): new insights into an old disease. Jama 283: 897–903
23. Sohn DW, Jung JW, Oh BH, et al (2001) Should ascending aortic intramural hematoma be treated surgically? Am J Cardiol 87: 1024–1026; A1025

Panel Discussion 2
What's New in Aortic Root Reimplantation?

What's New in Aortic Root Reimplantation?

The Valsalva Graft Design in its Anatomical Reconstruction of the Aortic Root

Ruggero De Paulis, Raffaele Scaffa, Daniele Maselli, Alessandro Bellisario, and Andrea Salica

Summary Valve-sparing operations for aortic root aneurysms are increasing in frequency, but techniques and results are still under evaluation. The aortic root is a dynamic unit that performs very sophisticated cyclic movements. Its dynamic characteristics are aimed at reducing stress on the cusps, and optimizing ventricular-arterial coupling to warrant hemodynamic efficiency without structural deterioration of the cusps over time. A better understanding of aortic valve function has led to appreciation of the role of adjacent structures in modulating leaflet movements. A very important step in this direction was the recognition of the role of the sinuses of Valsalva in smooth leaflet approximation. The reimplantation type of valve sparing procedure using the new Valsalva graft that incorporates the neo-sinuses, combines the advantages of proper anatomical reconstruction typical of the original remodeling technique with those of annular stabilization proper of the original reimplantation technique. The surgical approach and the various steps can be standardized and overall results are reproducible. Whether these improvements will translate in extending the long-term durability of the aortic leaflets remain to be determined.

Keywords remodeling · reimplantation · Valsava sinuses · aortic root · aortic aneurysm

Introduction

Sinotubular (ST) junction dilatation often due to ascending aortic aneurysm is one of the main cause of aortic valve regurgitation and can be simply treated by reducing the ST-junction at normal size using a Dacron conduit [1]. For many years in patients with ascending aortic aneurysm involving the sinuses of Valsalva associated with aortic incompetence the standard surgical therapy was the implantation of

---

R.D. Paulis (✉), R. Scaffa, D. Maselli, A. Bellisario, and A. Salica
Department of Cardiac Surgery. European Hospital, Via Portuense 700-00149-Rome, Italy
e-mail: depauli@tin.it

a valved conduit. In order to preserve the native valve, avoid life-long anticoagulation, and restore normal valve function by recreating a normal anatomic root, techniques of valve-sparing procedures have been developed. The importance of the sinuses of Valsalva in the aortic valve function has been debated since the time of Leonardo da Vinci [2]. A better understanding of aortic valve function is now gradually leading us to appreciation of the role of the adjacent structures in modulating leaflet movements. A very important step in this direction was the recognition of the role that the sinuses of Valsalva play in smooth leaflet approximation. Various dynamic factors cause the cusps to slowly approximate during late systole allowing the valve to close completely without any leaking closing volume and with low closing speed. Due to the eddy currents within the sinuses, the cusps start to slowly close before forward flow has ended; when blood flow reverses in diastole, remaining cusp excursion is small and valve closure is smooth with minimal stress and closing volume. Cyclic expansion of the sinuses contributes to a reduction of the systolic and diastolic stress on the valve leaflets and this stress sharing is important for the longevity of the aortic valve leaflets [3,4]. In fact, when the aortic root is replaced with less elastic artificial material the normal aortic root physiology may be lost, with impaired aortic valve opening and closing characteristics [5].

Valve-sparing Procedures

The Yacoub "remodelling" technique reduces the sinotubular junction and creates 3 neosinuses of Valsalva by using a scalloped Dacron tube in the supravalvular position [6]. David proposed the "reimplantation" of the aortic valve within a straight tube placed over the entire aortic root structure, reducing both the annulus and the sinotubular junction diameters [7]. The main difference between the two techniques is how the annulus is treated and whether the sinuses are preserved. The known advantages of the reimplantation technique like annulus stabilization, optimal support of the aortic wall and decreased chance for bleeding are reduced by the drawback of the complete lack of sinuses of Valsalva. In aortic root surgery, geometry and function of the complex unit of valve cusps and sinus of Valsalva are altered due to the unelastic graft wall and the lack of dynamic diameter changes. Leyh and colleagues found clinically that a more normal pattern of aortic valve dynamics and root distensibility might be better preserved with the remodelling technique compared with the reimplantation technique, supporting the hypothesis of better preserved valve function because of the presence of sinuses [8]. Recent publications have confirmed with direct imaging that in the standard reimplantation technique the preserved aortic valve showed bending and asymmetric motion. Conversely, in the remodelling technique, the preserved aortic valve opened and closed flexibly and symmetrically, similar to what was seen in the native aortic root [9].

From 1995 until today a series of technical variations have been proposed in order to overcome from the one side the lack of annulus stabilization and the risk of bleeding of the remodelling procedure and from other side the lack of sinuses of the reimplantation procedure. All of the techniques have evolved based upon an increased understanding of the functional anatomy of the aortic root complex.

In 1995 Dr. Cochran have modified the David procedure to produce an outward bulging sinus and a more natural environment for the aortic valve. To increase the proximal circumference of the conduit the graft was trimmed to create three symmetric scallops in the "annular" end of the Dacron conduit and then inserted (similar to the original technique described by David) with symmetric, subvalvular stitches along the annulus, followed by standard resuspension of the valve within the conduit [10].

However, over the time, Dr. David has frequently changed its own reimplantation technique utilizing a larger than needed prosthesis to provide redundant space at the sinus level. The "T. David-IV" (so-called in a recent editorial by Miller) is a reimplantation that uses a 4-mm larger graft size with circumferentially plication at the ST-junction above the tops of the commissures [11]. In the "T. David V" an oversized graft (6–8 mm larger than originally needed) is necked down proximally (annulus) and at the top ends (ST junction) to create graft pseudosinuses [12].

In 2004 Dr. Miller described a simple modification of the "T. David V" using 2 graft of different sizes (34-mm proximally and 24-mm graft distally) to create large pseudosinuses of Valsalva and a neo ST-junction [13]. Recently, Dr. Rama suggested another new original technique for aortic root inclusion [14]. Finally, Dr. Lansac and coll. suggested in the remodeling procedure the addiction of an external subvalvular prosthetic ring annuloplasty to prevent aortic insufficiency due to annular dilation [15].

In 2000 we introduced a new prosthesis that incorporates the sinuses of Valsalva (Gelweave Valsalva; Sulzer Vascutek, Renfrewshire, Scotland) [16]. Its main advantages are in a proper anatomical reconstruction of the aortic root while at the same time simplify the various steps and standardize the reimplantation type of valve sparing procedure, so reducing the importance of the surgeon experience and dexterity ("*less art than science*"). The original feature of this new Dacron graft is a short segment of the same material with corrugations parallel to the conduit long axis. This segment, called "the skirt", has a length equal to the graft diameter and is resilient in the horizontal plane so that, upon implantation and pressurization (it expands by 25–30% of its diameter), it will generate pseudosinuses of Valsalva. The suture joining these 2 sections of Dacron acts like a new sinotubular junction. For its intrinsic characteristics the Valsalva design provides an optimal anatomical aortic root reconstruction. In fact, the normal ST junction is slightly larger than the aortic annulus and the size ratio is 1.3 to 1 in a human adult heart [17]. In a normal aortic root the average leaflet height is similar to the average sinus height and the average coaptation height is right in the centre of the aortic root [18]. The Valsalva graft provides a normal proportion of component because the graft has, by design, a proportion of 1:1 between the annulus and the ST junction.

Furthermore, given the importance of the sinuses of Valsalva for a long-lasting leaflets function, with the use of the Valsalva graft design several goals can be achieved: a proper proportion of the various root components; a preserved an clear entrance of the blood flow into the sinuses; a preserved egg-like shape of the sinuses; and a certain degree of distensibility at the level of the sinuses [19]. It goes without saying that achieving all these goals helps the surgeon to avoid suboptimal leaflet coaptation that may result in early failure of the repair. In fact, Harringer and associates showed that patients with poor geometrical leaflet coaptation and greater than grade I aortic insufficiency had a high rate of reoperation [20].

Procedure Simplification

Our technique follows the steps described by David. Cardiopulmonary bypass is usually instituted through cannulation of the right atrium and the ascending aorta or aortic arch. Once the cardioplegia is administered, the ascending aorta is transacted and the aortic valve exposed. The external aspect of the aortic wall at the level of each commissure is dissected free from the right ventricular outflow tract (LVOT), from the pulmonary artery, and from the wall of both atria. This is necessary in order to facilitate placement of the subannular stitches later in the procedure. All three sinuses of Valsalva are excised, leaving a limited part of the arterial wall (3–5 mm) attached to the aortic valve and a small button of arterial wall around the left and right coronary arteries. As already stated, and confirmed by aortic valve sparing literature, a proper relationship between aortic valve annulus and ST-junction diameter is an important factor in aortic valve function. A considerable number of attempts to define standard rules for selection of the correct sizing of the Dacron conduit have been made in the last several years. It is usually predetermined on the basis of experience or intraoperative mathematical calculations [21–24]. We suggest the intraoperative measurement of the internal aortic annular diameter, as the sole criterion determining the choice of the prosthetic tube graft. In fact, after sizing the annulus we add 5 mm to obtain the conduit optimal size (e.g. for a 25 mm choose a 30 mm Valsalva graft). Recently, these findings were also confirmed by an in-vitro experimental settings using direct endoscopic view and ultrasound imaging techniques [25]. Multiple interrupted horizontal pledgeted mattress sutures are then passed from inside to outside the left ventricular outflow tract immediately below the aortic valve in a horizontal plane starting from the interleaflet triangles. When using the Valsalva graft, an important step is to adapt the height of the skirt to the height of the patients commissures in order to obtain a correct placement of the top of the commissures at the level of the union of the skirted section and the standard graft which represents the new ST junction. This is achieved by sizing the height of the commissures from the annular stitches to the top of the commissure and reporting this measure to the skirt of the prosthesis. In case of perfect correspondence between the length of the skirt and the height of the commissures, the sub-annular U-stitches are placed on the Dacron graft right at the base of the skirt. When the height of the commissures are shorter than the skirt, the skirt can be trimmed at the proper level or alternatively the first row of suture are passed at the proper distance from the base of the skirt. The valve is then retrieved from inside and the valve remnants are suture to the graft. Finally, coronary buttons and distal graft sutures complete the procedure.

Procedure Standardization and Reproducibility

The use of aortic valve-sparing operations has increased in the last years owing to a better understanding of anatomy, function and pathology of the aortic root. Since 2000, the Gelweave Valsalva graft has been available to facilitate the creation of sinuses of Valsalva of normal shape and dimension. The Italian experience of three cardiac surgery departments in the reimplantation type of valve-sparing procedure using this conduit was analyzed in the clinical results of the first 151 patients. In this paper at 5 years, freedom from aortic valve replacement and freedom from grade 3 to 4 aortic insufficiency was 90.8% ± 3.3% and 88.7% ± 3.6%, respectively [26].

A retrospective review was also performed on 35 patients with Marfan syndrome who underwent the reimplantation valve-sparing aortic root replacement using the Gelweave Valsalva prosthesis in four different centres. Significant aortic insufficiency, requiring aortic valve replacement, developed in 3 patients during follow-up. The 5-year freedom from reoperation owing to structural valve deterioration was 88.9% ± 8.1% [27]. Criticism of the Valsalva conduit has centred on the predetermined height of the sinus segment [13]. However, in this review of patients with Marfan syndrome, the graft size distribution (1 pts: 26 mm; 11 pts: 28 mm; 14 pts: 30 mm and 9 pts: 32 mm) demonstrate that none of the patients had aortic valve commissures that exceeded 3.5 cm or more, which would exceed the height of the skirt in the Valsalva graft.

Finally, excellent results have been reported by the use of the Valsalva graft in a large pediatric population. Most of the patients were Marfan and the reported freedom from residual aortic regurgitation was 100 % at 1, 8 years [28].

An ongoing registry is available at www.valsalvaregistry.com for all users that would like to contribute in collecting a large series to evaluate the long-term durability of valve leaflet after a reimplantation type of valve sparing procedure using the Valsalva graft.

Conclusions

The reimplantation technique for valve sparing procedure has become the most frequently used technique because it guarantees more stable results in the long-term period when compared to the remodelling technique. However, even though medium term results of the standard technique are promising [29] the lack of sinuses of Valsalva, typical of this procedure, has cast doubts over the long-term durability of the valve cusps. In the recent years, a great number of technical variations to the standard surgical technique have been described, mainly with the scope of re-creating the sinuses of Valsalva. All these techniques require a certain degree of technical skill and a good tridimensional view of the aortic root. In this respect, the Valsalva graft offers the possibility of following the usual standard steps of the original technique as first described by David. As a direct consequence, the procedure can be easily standardized and reproduced and at the same time an optimal anatomical root reconstruction can be readily achieved. If a perfect morphological root reconstruction will extend the life span of the spared aortic leaflets remains to be determined.

References

1. David TE, Feindel CM, Armstrong S, et al (2007) Replacement of the ascending aorta with reduction of the diameter of the sinotubular junction to treat aortic insufficiency in patients with ascending aortic aneurysm. J Thorac Cardiovasc Surg 133:414–8
2. Morea M, De Paulis R (2007) "Il buso" (the orifice) How much did Leonardo know of the aortic valve?. J Cardiovasc Med 8:399–403
3. Kunzelman KS, Grande J, David TE, et al (1994) Aortic root and valve relationships: Impact on surgical repair. J Thorac Cardiovasc Surg 107:162–170
4. Kvitting JP, Ebbers T, Wigstrom L, et al (2004) Flow patterns in the aortic root and the aorta studied with time-resolved, 3-dimensional, phase-contrast magnetic resonance imaging: implications for aortic valve-sparing surgery J Thorac Cardiovasc Surg 127:1602–1607
5. Robicsek F, Thubrikar MJ, Fokin AA (2002) Cause of degenerative disease of the trileaflet aortic valve: review of subject and presentation of a new theory. Ann Thorac Surg 73:1346–54
6. Sarsam MA, Yacoub M (1993) Remodeling of the aortic valve anulus. J Thorac Cardiovasc Surg 105:435–8
7. David TE, Feindel CM (1992) An aortic valve-sparing operation for patients with aortic incompetence and aneurysm of the ascending aorta. J Thorac Cardiovasc Surg 103:617–22
8. Leyh RG, Schmidtke C, Sievers HH, et al (1999) Opening and closing characteristics of the aortic valve after different types of valve-preserving surgery. Circulation 100:2153–60
9. Furukawa K, Ohteki H, Cao ZL, et al (2004) Evaluation of native valve-sparing aortic root reconstruction with direct imaging- reimplantation or remodeling? Ann Thorac Surg 77:1636–41
10. Cochran RP, Kunzelman KS, Eddy AC, et al (1995) Modified conduit preparation creates a pseudosinus in an aortic valve–sparing procedure for aneurysm of the ascending aorta. J Thorac Cardiovasc Surg 109:1049–1058
11. David TE, Armstrong S, Ivanov J, et al (2001) Results of aortic valve-sparing operations. J Thorac Cardiovasc Surg 122:39–46
12. de Oliveira NC, David TE, Ivanov J, et al (2003) Results of surgery for aortic root aneurysm in patients with Marfan syndrome J Thorac Cardiovasc Surg 125:789–796
13. Demers P, Miller DC (2004) Simple modification of "T. David V" valve-sparing aortic root replacement to create graft psudosinuses. Ann Thorac Surg 78:1479–81
14. Rama A, Rubin S, Bonnet N, et al (2007) New technique of aortic root reconstruction with aortic valve annuloplasty in ascending aortic aneurysm. Ann Thorac Surg 83:1908–1910
15. Lansac E, Di Centa I, Bonnet N, et al (2006) Aortic prosthetic ring annuloplasty: a useful adjunct to a standardized aortic valve-sparing procedure? Eur J Cardiothorac Surg 29:537–544
16. De Paulis R, De Matteis GM, Nardi P, et al (2000) A new aortic Dacron conduit for surgical treatment of aortic root pathology. Ital Heart J 1:457–63
17. Acar C. 6th Symposium on aortic and mitral reconstructive surgery. Brussels 2006
18. Vijay V et al. EACTS/ESTS Joint Meeting 2000 (abstract)
19. De Paulis R, De Matteis GM, Nardi P, et al (2002) Analysis of valve motion after the reimplantation type of valve-sparing procedure (David I) with a new aortic root conduit. Ann Thorac Surg 74:53–57
20. Pethig K, Milz A, Hagl C, et al (2002) Aortic valve reimplantation in ascending aortic aneurysm: risk factors for early valve failure. Ann Thorac Surg 73:29–33

21. David TE, Ivanon J, Armstrong S, et al (2002) Aortic valve-sparing operations in patients with aneurysm of the aortic root or ascending aorta. Ann Thorac Surg 74:S1758–61
22. Svensson LG (2003) Sizing for modified David's reimplantation procedure. Ann Thorac Surg 76:1751–3
23. Hopkins RA (2003) Aortic valve leaflet sparing and salvage surgery: evolution of techniques for aortic root reconstruction. Eur J Cardiothorac Surg 24:886–97
24. Gleason TG (2005) New graft formulation and modification of the David reimplantation technique. J Thorac Cardiovasc Surg 130:601–3
25. Maselli D, De Paulis R, Scaffa R, et al (2007) Sinotubuluar junction size affects aortic root geometry and aortic valve function in the aortic valve reimplantation procedure: an in vitro study using the Valsalva graft. Ann Thorac Surg 84:1214–8
26. Pacini D, Settepani F, De Paulis R, et al (2006) Early results of valve-sparing reimplantation procedure using the Valsalva conduit: A multicenter study. Ann Thorac Surg 82:865–872
27. Settepani F, Szeto WY, Pacini D, et al (2007) Reimplantation valve-sparing aortic root replacement in Marfan syndrome using the Valsalva conduit: an intercontinental multicenter study. Ann Thorac Surg 83:S769–S773
28. Patel ND, Williams JA, Barreiro CJ, et al (2006) Valve-Sparing Aortic Root Replacement: Early Experience With the De Paulis Valsalva Graft in 51 Patients. Ann Thorac Surg 82:548–553
29. Kallenbach K, Baraki H, Khaladj N, et al (2007) Aortic Valve–Sparing Operation in Marfan Syndrome: What Do We Know After a Decade? Ann Thorac Surg 83:S764–S768

Expanding Indications for Valve Sparing Procedures in Aortic Root Replacement

Yutaka Okita, Masamichi Matsumori, Kenji Okada,
Yoshihisa Morimoto, Mitsuru Asano, Hiroshi Munakata,
Naoto Morimoto, Hiroaki Takahashi, and Akiko Tanaka

Summary From October 1999 to December 2007, 61 patients with annulo-aortic ectasia underwent aortic root replacement with aortic cusp sparing procedure. The mean age was 48.7 ± 15.1 years old and there were 42 male and 19 females. Preoperative aortic regurgitation was measured as none in 6, grade 1 in 11, grade 2 in 8, grade 3 in 20, and grade 4 in 16. Twenty patients had Marfan syndrome, 11 had acute aortic dissection, and 1 had Takayasu's aortitis. Root remodeling procedure was performed in only one patient with aortic monocuspid valve and the other 60 patients had the reimplantation technique. Initial 12 patients had a straight Dacron graft for aortic root. Since July 2002, the bulging-sinus graft (22 hand-made and 26 DePaulis's anteflo Vaskteck graft) was used. Repair techniques for abnormal aortic cusps consisted with plication of the free margins at the Arantius body (15 patients), reinforcement of the free margin of the cusp (5), patch plasty using the autologous pericardium (3), and plication at the commissure (2). The size of the implanted Dacron graft was 24 mm (9), 26 mm (45), and 28 mm (7). Simultaneous surgery consisted with total arch replacement in 12 patients, hemiarch replacement in 6, mitral valve repair in 3, Maze procedure in 2, axillo-femoral bypass in 1 and repair of aortic coarctation in 2. [Results] There no early and late death. Echocardiogram 1 month after surgery disclosed that aortic regurgitation was none (26), grade I (29), and grade II (6). During hospitalization, 2 patients required reoperation because of residual or recurrent aortic regurgitation. Follow-up was 41.8 ± 10.6 months, ranging 2 months to 8.4 yrs. Echocardiogram at latest follow-up demonstrated that aortic regurgitation was none (15), grade I (18), grade II (3), grade III (1), and grade IV (2) and 2 patients required reoperation

---

Y. Okita, M. Matsumori, K. Okada, Y. Morimoto, M. Asano, H. Munakata, N. Morimoto,
H. Takahashi, and A. Tanaka
Division of Cardiovascular Surgery, Department of Surgery
Kobe University Graduate School of Medicine, Kobe, Japan

Y. Okita (✉)
Division of Cardiovascular Surgery, Department of Surgery
Kobe University Graduate School of Medicine, Kobe, Japan
7-5-2 Kusunoki-cho, Chuo-ku, Kobe, Hyogo, Japan 650-0017
e-mail: yokita@med.kobe-u.ac.jp

because of aortic regurgitation. Freedom from the reoperation in patients who had additional aortic cusp repairs was similar to the patients who had simple aortic reimplantation. Also freedom from significant aortic regurgitation (more than grade II) in patients with cusp repair was not different from that of patients without cusp repair. Regarding the techniques of aortic cusp repair, patients who had placation at the commissure (Trusler) tended to have worse outcome compared with patients who had other repair techniques, such as patch closure of the defects, placation at the Arantius body, and reinforcement of the free margin. Similary the diameter of sinus Valsalva over 50 mm, coexistence of the acute aortic dissection has no correlations to the postoperative aortic regurgitation. [Conclusion] Indications of valve sparing aortic root replacement have been expanded. Minor abnormalities of the cusps, such as prolapse, fenestrations, and stretched free margin, did not excluded cusp sparing and mid-term results of the cusp repairing procedure was comparable with the simple cusp sparing root replacement.

Keywords Aortic root replacement · reimplantation · aortic valve repair

Introduction

The gold standard for replacing the aortic root has still been the Bentall-DeBono operation since 1968 [1], however, complications related to the anticoagulation and structural or non-structural prosthesis deterioration have shifted the paradigm towards the valve sparing aortic root operation, such as Yacoub's remodeling [2] and David's reimplantation [3] procedures. A certain amount of patients has normal aortic cusp with dilatation of left ventricular outflow tract (basal ring), sinus of Valsalva and sino-tubular junction (ST junction). These patients can have the most benefit of the valve sparing operation.

Recent debate over the superiority of the two procedures has almost reached conclusions [4]. The future dilatation of the basal ring and interleaflet triangle after remodeling operation has precluded application of the remodeling procedure to the young Marfan patients with dilated basal ring. Patients with less enlargement of the basal ring with dilatation of the sinus and ST junction usually tolerate the remodeling procedure. The intrinsic disadvantage of the reimplantation procedure is theoretically considered to be that the straight Dacron tube has no physiological effects of the sinus Valsalva. Although numerous modifications of the reimplantation to mimic the Valsalva sinus has been tried, such as those of Cochran [5], DePaulis graft [6], David V operation [4], Stanford [7] and Gleason [8], none has could demonstrated the advantages of hemodynamic and long-term durability over the straight graft clinically. Another challenge in this field has been tried in repairing the abnormal aortic cusps. Cusp prolapse is often seen in this patient population. Several techniques, such as plication or reinforcement of the stretched free margin, and patching the defect have been applied. But also the valve sparing root procedures has be en applied in patients with acute aortic dissection. The long-term results in these patients have not been yet proven.

In this paper, our experience of the aortic root replacement with valve sparing procedure has been described with underscoring the cusp repairing technique.

Patients

From October 1999 to December 2007, we have completed aortic root replacement with aortic cusp sparing procedure in 61 patients with annulo-aortic ectasia. During the same periods, initial plan for the valve sparing was changed to the Bentall's operation after observing the aortic cusps in 11 patients with annulo-aortic ectasia. Intraoperative conversion after finishing the valve sparing procedure to the Bentall's operation was necessary in another 2 patients. The mean age was 48.7 ± 15.1 years old and there were 42 male and 19 females. Emergency surgery was performed because of acute dissection in 11 patients. Preoperative NYHA functional class was I in 45, II in 5, III & IV in zero in elective patients. Preoperative aortic regurgitation was measured as none in 6, grade 1 in 11, grade 2 in 8, grade 3 in 20, and grade 4 in 16 (Fig. 1). The dimensions of the aortic root were presented in the Table 1. Twenty patients had Marfan syndrome, 11 had acute aortic dissection, and 1 had Takayasu's aortitis. As for acute type A aortic dissection, aortic root replacement was performed when the tear was found in the Valsalva sinus or when the patients have pre-existing annuloaortic ectasia. There were 4 patients with the bicuspid aortic valve and one with monocusp. Ten patients, including one with Ross procedure, had a previous aortic root surgery.

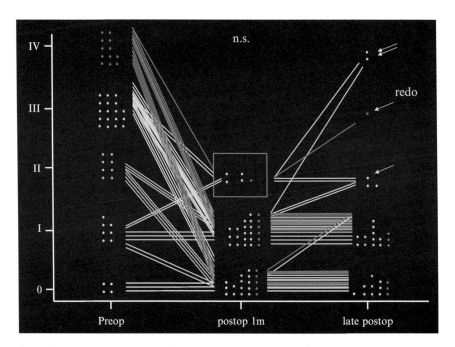

Fig. 1 Cusp repair. Free margin plication at the Arantius body using 7–0 Prolene

Table 1 Cardio-aortic dimensions

	Preop	postop	follow-up
Dd	55.2 ± 8.2	45.8 ± 4.5	47.8 ± 4.8
Ds	37.8 ± 7.8	36.6 ± 8.4	32.3 ± 5.1
%FS	33.9 ± 8.1	27.2 ± 9.2	35.1 ± 9.4
LVOT	26.1 ± 3.1	19.2 ± 1.8	20.4 ± 3.1
Sinus	47.8 ± 7.5	29.9 ± 3.4	29.8 ± 2.5
ST junction	24.9 ± 4.2	23.3 ± 1.7	25.55 ± 2.8

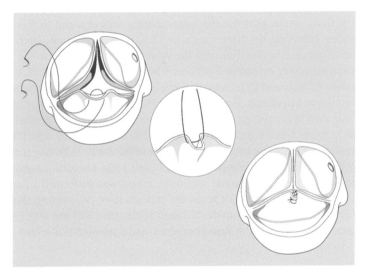

Fig. 2 Managing fenestrations. Reinforcement of the free margin. Excluding the fenestration using CV-7 Gore-Tex suture in 2 rows, tying outside the aorta

Root remodeling procedure was performed in only one patient with aortic monocuspid valve and the other 60 patients had the reimplantation technique. Initial 12 patients had a straight Dacron graft for aortic root. Since July 2002, the bulging-sinus graft (22 hand-made and 26 DePaulis's anteflo Vaskteck graft) was used. Several repair techniques for abnormal aortic cusps were applied. Plication of the free margins for several millimeters at the Arantius body using 6–0 or 7–0 polypropylene suture (Prolene) was applied in 15 patients who had prolapsed aortic cusps (Fig. 2). Reinforcement of the free margin of the cusp using 7–0 EPTFE suture (Gore-Tex) was applied in 5 patients with large fenestrations of the cusp, where the remained free margin was so friable like a chord (Fig. 3). For larger fenestrations or cusp defect, patch plasty using the autologous pericardium in 3 patients (Fig. 4). Plication at the commissure [9] was performed in 2 patients. In patients with acute type A aortic dissection, the dissected layers with the GRF glue were fixed and then the sinus wall was scalloped (Fig. 5). The size of the implanted Dacron graft was 24 in 9 patients, 26 in 45, and 28 in 7. Simultaneous surgery consisted with total arch replacement in 12 patients, hemiarch replacement in 6, mitral valve repair in 3, Maze procedure in 2, axillo-femoral bypass in 1 and repair of aortic coarctation in 2.

Expanding Indications for Valve Sparing Procedures in Aortic Root Replacement 177

Fig. 3 Managing larger fenestrations. Closure of the defect using an autologous pericardial patch

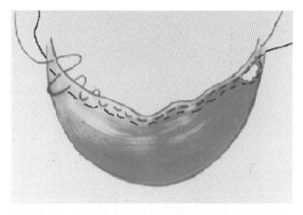

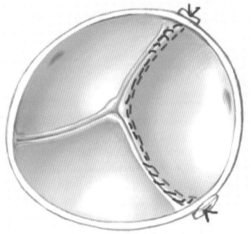

Fig. 4 Transition of the severity of aoric regurgitatioin according to the preop AR grade

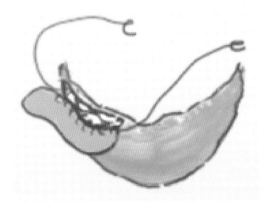

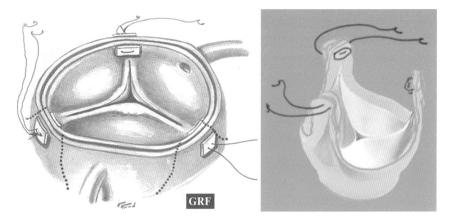

Fig. 5 Managing acute dissection complicated with annuloaortic ectasia. The commissurewas fixed with the GRF glueand then scalloping the Valsalva sinus was performed

Results

No early death was encountered. Total cardiopulmonary bypass time and cardiac ischemic time was 229 ± 49 (154 – 348) minutes and 177 ± 32 (123 – 289) minutes respectively. A few perioperative morbidities were found, such as bleeding necessitating reoperation in 2 patients and complete AV block in 1. There were no patients who had heart failure, respiratory failure, and renal failure. Echocardiogram 1 month after surgery disclosed that aortic regurgitation was none in 26 patients, grade I in 29, grade II in 6, no grade III and grade IV patients. During hospitalization, 2 patients required reoperation because of residual or recurrent aortic regurgitation. One was 53 old male who had Ross procedure for para-annular aortic abscess 3 years before developed severe neo-aortic regurgitation. Aortic reimplantation using a home-made Valsalva graft (26 mm Intergard woven Dacron graft) and plication of the left coronary cusp was performed. However, progressive deterioration of the aortic regurgitation was noticed and he underwent aortic valve replacement with a mechanical prosthesis one month later. The other patient was 55 year-old male with acute type A aortic dissection who underwent an emergency surgery. Aortic root was grossly dilated and a large intimal tear was found in the ascending aorta. A simple aortic reimplantation using a 26 mm DePaulis' graft and hemiarch replacement was performed. Although residual aortic regurgitation was mild, intractable hemolysis due to the mechanical shear stress necessitated replacement of the aortic valve with a mechanical prosthesis two months later. The Cardio-aortic dimension at discharge was listed in table 1. During follow-up of 41.8 ± 10.6 months, ranging 2 months to 8.4 yrs, no late deaths was observed. Echocardiogram at latest follow-up demonstrated that aortic regurgitation was none in 15 patients, grade I in 18, grade II in 3, grade III in 1, and grade IV in 2 patients (Fig. 1). Two patients required reoperation because of aortic regurgitation. One was 51 old female with aortitis syndrome and she developed annulo-aortic ectasia and aortic arch aneurysm. She underwent aortic root reimplantation and total arch replacement. Early postoperative echocardiogram showed no aortic regurgitation, however, gradual increase of the regurgitation ensued and she finally had aortic valve replacement 2 years later. At reoperation, fibrosed and retracted aortic cusps were documented and valve was replaced with a mechanical prosthesis. The other reoperated patient was 54 year-old female with Marfan syndrome. She had aortic root reimplantation with home-made Valsalva graft. Aortic cusps were elongated and left coronary cusp was prolapsed. Trsuler type cusp placation stitches were placed at the both end of the free margin at each commissure of the left coronary cusp, however, immediately postoperative echo demonstrated mild to moderate aortic regurgitation. One year later, aortic valve replacement was performed with a mechanical prosthesis.

Freedom from the reoperation in patients who had additional aortic cusp repairs was similar to the patients who had simple aortic reimplantation (Fig. 6). Also freedom from significant aortic regurgitation (more than grade II) in patients with cusp repair was not different from that of patients without cusp repair (Fig. 7). Regarding the techniques of aortic cusp repair, patients who had placation at the commissure (Trusler) tended to have worse outcome compared with patients who had other repair techniques, such as patch closure of the defects, placation at the Arantius body, and reinforcement of the free margin. (Fig. 8). Regarding the preoperative diameter of sinus Valsalva over 50 mm and coexistence of the acute aortic dissection, postoperative aortic regurgitation has no correlation to them (Fig. 9 and 10).

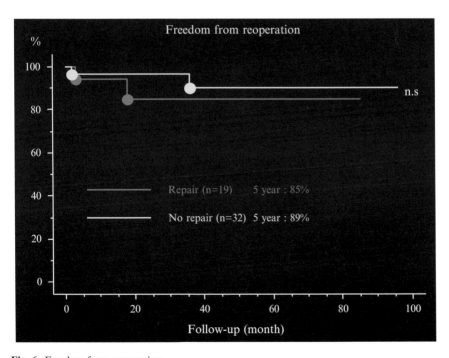

Fig. 6 Freedom from reoperation

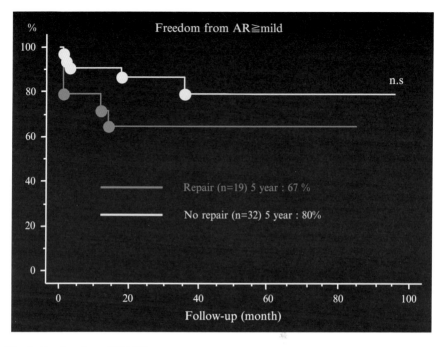

Fig. 7 Freedom from AR ≥ 2/4

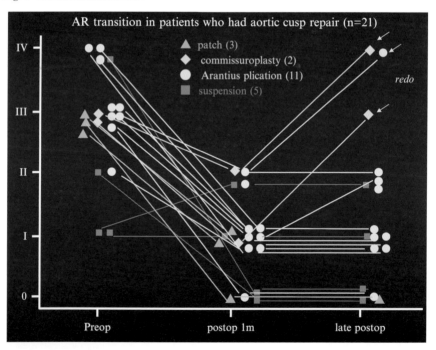

Fig. 8 Transition of the severity of aoric regurgitatioin according to the various cusp reapir technique

Expanding Indications for Valve Sparing Procedures in Aortic Root Replacement

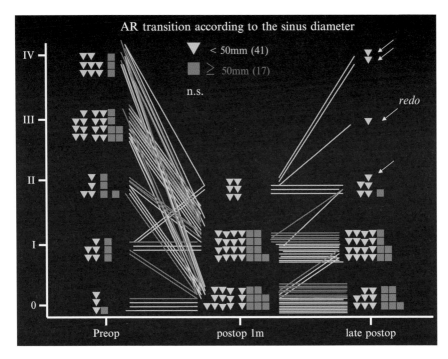

Fig. 9 Transition of the severity of aoric regurgitatioin according to the sinus diameter

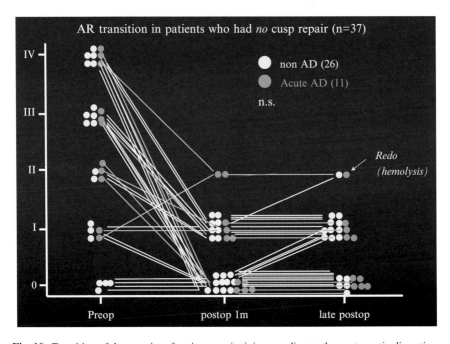

Fig. 10 Transition of the severity of aoric regurgitatioin according to the acute aortic dissection

Discussion

Establishment of surgical repair techniques for mitral valve regurgitation has promoted a clinical application of "analogue" strategies in aortic valve repair. However, not many studies regarding aortic valve repair have been reported except for congenitally bicuspid aortic valve disease [10] or rheumatic aortic valve disease [11]. On the other hand, aortic valve replacement using mechanical valve or biological valve was technically reproducible and brought excellent early-postoperative homodynamic. Initially the long-term results of simple aortic valve replacement was believed to be satisfactory, however, clinical accumulation of the long-term results disclosed that significant numbers of premature deterioration of the prosthetic valve, anticoagulation-related hemorrhage or thromboembolism, and non-structural valve dysfunction have set limitation in survival of the patients [12,13].

Pathological studies and clinical experiences disclosed that aortic cusps in patients with annulo-aortic ectasia usually show normal structure or minimum abnormalities. The gold standard for replacing the aortic root is still the Bentall-DeBono operation [1] in the present time, however, novel technical expertise's such as Yacoub's remodeling [2] or David's reimplantation [3] procedures have gained a increasing popularity in the surgical strategies for patients with annul aortic ectasia.

Minimum requirement for the aortic root replacement with valve sparing technique was initially "structurally normal aortic cusps" [2], however, recent advancement of knowledge regarding physiology of the aortic root and refinement of the surgical technique have enabled concomitant repair of the aortic cusp and reconstruction of the aortic root [4].

There are many reasons regarding residual or recurrent aortic regurgitation in patients who underwent aortic cusp sparing root replacement. Most clear reasons are preoperative failure to set the proper indications of this procedure, such as gross calcified cusps, thickened or shrunk cusps, and over stretched cusps. However, not a few patients had recurrent regurgitation due to surgery-related postoperative cusp prolapse. This iatrogenic cusp prolapse usually developed due to uneven annular reduction and malposition of the commissure, horizontally or vertically. Sometimes suture-cutting trauma of the cusp leads to early reoperation. During follow-up, annular dilatation, which is intrinsically defect of the remodeling procedure, cusp traumatism due to the hitting the graft, cusp disease development in the connective tissue disease, and endocarditis are possible causes for reoperation.

Cusp prolapse is often seen in this patient population and the etiology of this prolapse was thought to be rupture of the fragile chord at the fenestration of the cusps [14]. Several techniques, such as plication of the free margin at the Arantius body, triangular resection and sutures of the Arantius body, or plicating the free margin at the commissure (Trusler) were reported but resection and suture technique and Trusler's technique usually show premature failures during follow-up. Cusp fenestration near the free margin itself is not responsible for valvular regurgitation, however, we are concerned that possible rupture of a finite chord-like structure at the cusp free margin may result in cusp prolapse. Reinforcement of the free margin using a double row of Gore-Tex sutures (CV-7) have been tried in this setting but no long-term results was reported yet. Moreover, this technique has potential risks for damaging the cusp. For larger fenestrations, we sometimes close the defect using glutaraldehyde-treated autologous pericardium.

During repair of acute type A aortic dissection, aortic root replacement is required when the tear was found in the Valsalva sinus, or the sinus was destroyed and when the patients have pre-existing annuloaortic ectasia. Several promising reports [15] encouraged us to apply the valve sparing root replacement in the setting of acute type A dissection. Secure fixation of the intimo-media and adventitia tissue at the commissure is mandatory to have competent valve. We use GRF glue in the false lumen but tissue necrosis due to formalin is some concern.

We found no statistically significant difference regarding the freedom from the mild or more aortic regurgitation and incidence of reoperation between the patients who had cusp repair or without. Also preoperative severity of the aortic regurgitation, size of the Valsalva sinus, and presence of the acute aortic dissection has no correlation to postoperative severity of the residual or recurrent valve regurgitation.

Conclusion

Indications of valve sparing aortic root replacement have been expanded. Minor abnormalities of the cusps, such as prolapse, fenestrations, and stretched free margin, did not excluded cusp sparing and mid-term results of the cusp repairing procedure was comparable with the simple cusp sparing root replacement.

References

1. Bentall H, De Bono A (1968) A technique for complete replacement of the ascending aorta. Thorax 23:338–339
2. Sarsam MA, Yacoub M (1993) Remodeling of the aortic valve anulus. J Thorac Cardiovasc Surg 105:435–438
3. David TE, Ivanov J, Armstrong S, et al (2002) Aortic valve-sparing operations in patients with aneurysms of the aortic root or ascending aorta. Ann Thorac Surg 74:S1758–761
4. David TE, Feindel CM, Webb GD, et al (2007) Long-term results of aortic valve–sparing operations for aortic root aneurysm. J Thorac Cardiovasc Surg 132:347–54
5. Cochran RP, Kunzelman KS, Eddy AC, et al (1995) Modified conduit preparation creates a pseudosinus in an aortic valve-sparing procedure for aneurysm of the ascending aorta. J Thorac Cardiovasc Surg 109:1049–1057
6. De Paulis R, Bassano C, Scaffa R, et al (2004) Bentall procedures with a novel valved conduit incorporating "sinuses of Valsalva". Surg Technol Int 12:195–200
7. Demers P, Miller DC (2004) Simple modification of "T. David-V" valve-sparing aortic root replacement to create graft pseudosinuses. Ann Thorac Surg 78:1479–1481

8. Gleason TG (2006)Aortic annuloplasty and valve-sparing root replacement: details of the primary suture line. J Thorac Cardiovasc Surg 131:502–503
9. Trusler GA, Moes CAF, Kidd BSL (1973) Repair of ventricular septal defect with aortic insufficiency. J Thorac Cardiovasc Surg 66:394–403
10. Nash PJ, Vitvitsky E, Li J, et al (2005) Feasibility of Valve Repair for Regurgitant Bicuspid Aortic Valves - An Echocardiographic Study Ann Thorac Surg 79:1473–9
11. Duran C, Kumar N, Gometza B, et al (1991) Indications and limitations of aortic valve reconstruction. Ann Thorac Surg 52:447–54
12. Zellner JL, Kratz JM, Crumbley AJ 3rd, et al (1999) Long-term experience with the St. Jude Medical valve prosthesis. Ann Thorac Surg 68:1210–8
13. Jamieson WR, Janusz MT, MacNab J, et al (2001) Hemodynamic comparison of second- and third-generation stented bioprostheses in aortic valve replacement. Ann Thorac Surg 71:S282–4
14. De Waroux JB, Pouleur AC, Goffinet C, et al (2007) Functional anatomy of aortic regurgitation: accuracy, prediction of surgical repairability, and outcome implications of transesophageal echocardiography. Circulation 116:1264–9
15. Kallenbach K, Leyh RG, Salcher R, et al (2004) Acute aortic dissection versus aortic root aneurysm: comparison of indications for valve sparing aortic root reconstruction. Eur J Cardio-thorac Surg 25:663–70

Poster Session 1
Aortic Dissection, Marfan Syndrome

Sivelestat Sodium is Effective to Prevent Acute Lung Injury in Acute Aortic Dissection

Yasushige Shingu, Norihiko Shiiya, Suguru Kubota, Yuji Naito, Kinya Matsui, Satoru Wakasa, Hiroshi Sugiki, Tsuyoshi Tachibana, Tomoji Yamakawa, Toshifumi Murashita, and Yoshiro Matsui

Acute lung injury is a frequent and serious complication in patients with acute aortic dissection (AAD). Elevated neutrophil elastase has been reported to be one of the major contributing factots. We evaluated the effects of sivelestat sodium hydrate, a neutrophil elastase inhibitor, to prevent lung injury in medically treated patients with acute aortic dissection. Clinical course of eleven patients who received prophylactic sivelestat sodium hydrate was compared with that of twelve patients without it (control group). Although mechanical ventilation was required in four (42%) control group patients, none needed intubation in the sivelestat group. Our study suggested that sivelestat sodium hydrate might be effective to prevent respiratory failure in acute aortic dissection.

Y. Shingu, N. Shiiya, S. Kubota, Y. Naito, K. Matsui, S. Wakasa, H. Sugiki, T. Tachibana, T. Yamakawa, T. Murashita, and Y. Matsui
Department of Cardiovascular Surgery, Hokkaido University, Sapporo, Japan

Long-Term Results of Emergency Prosthetic Vascular Graft Replacement for Acute Stanford A Aortic Dissection

Sunao Watanabe, Kohei Abe, Manabu Yamazaki, Kazufumi Ohmori, and Hitoshi Koyanagi

From Jul/1997 to Jun/2007 65 patients (mean age 61; 31 to 87 years) underwent emergency graft replacement of the proximal aorta for acute Stanford A dissection.

Operative Method: Unless intimal tear was present in the arch, ascending aortic replacement was performed. As regards Valsalva sinus, we made effort as much as we could to appose intima and adventitia using GRF glue to reconstruct the structure and subsequently anastomose a tube graft to the transected proximal stump at the level just above the sino-tubular junction. Consequently, operative procedures in these 65 patients were: ascending replacement, 36; ascending to hemiarch, 7; valve-sparing root replacement, 2; Bentall, 11; total arch, 9.

Results: There were 2 operative deaths due to LMT occlusion (3.1%), and 2 other late hospital deaths. The remaining 61 were followed up with a mean period of 41 months. Survival rate of these patients at 10 years was 86%. There were 9 second operations (14.8%). Bentall procedure was done in 5, total arch replacement in 4, Bentall plus total arch in 1. Operative mortality in redo surgery was 1 in 9 (11.1%).

Conclusions: Emergency grafting for acute D/A could be performed with low operative mortality and satisfactory long-term survival rate.

Keywords aortic dissection · emergency surgery · long-term results · graft replacement · GRF glue

---

S. Watanabe, K. Abe, M. Yamazaki, K. Ohmori, and H. Koyanagi
Department of Cardiovascular Surgery, Heart Center,
St. Luke's International Hospital
9-1 Akashi-Cho, Chuo-Ku, Tokyo, 104-8560, Japan

S. Watanabe (✉)
St. Luke's International Hospital
e-mail: suwtnb@luke.or.jp

Operative Method

For onset-phase acute Stanford A aortic dissection, we have made it a strategy not to replace the aortic root, not to replace aortic arch, and replace only tubular portion of ascending aorta, unless there is an intimal tear in either aortic root or arch is present.

In aortic root, pseudolumen is obliterated with the use of Gelatin-Resorsin-Formalin (GRF) glue, and the stump is reinforced with Teflon felt strips applied both inside and around. For distal stump, the same reinforcement is applied before anastomosing the prosthetic tube graft under selective cerebral perfusion and trunkal circulatory arrest at the temperature of approximately 23°C.

Patients

Between Jul/1997 and Jun/2007, we have experienced 65 patients (mean age 61.0±13.4, 31 to 87 years old; male:female = 39:26; Marfan syndrome 5 (7.7%)) with onset-phase acute Stanford A aortic dissection for whom emergency surgery was performed. As a result of the minimal surgery strategy described above, more than half of these 65 patients (36 patients) underwent only ascending aortic replacement. Arch replacement was performed in 16 patients, and root replacement in 13 patients (Bentall op, 11; valve-sparing root replacement, 2).

Results

There were 2 operative deaths (3.1%) due to left main coronary trunk involvement with cardiogenic shock. Two additional patients with ascending aortic replacement died in late hospitalization period due to graft infection and septicemia. Remaining 61 patients were followed up with a mean period of 41±33 months (from 3 to 120 months).

Kaplan-Meier method showed the actuarial survival rate at 10-year point to be 86% (Fig.1a).

No statistically significant difference existed in terms of late survival rate among the groups who underwent ascending replacement only, arch replacement, and root replacement (Fig.1b). On the other hand, late survival rate was significantly less in patients who underwent redo aortic surgery, as compared with those who did not need additional intervention. (Fig.1c)

Discussion

- Emergency grafting for acute D/A could be performed with the mortality rate of 3.2%.
- Low mortality (as judged from the Japanese standard of 11.7% (hospital mortality) shown in the annual review [1]) could be attributed to the "minimal

Long-Term Results of Emergency Surgery for Type A Dissection

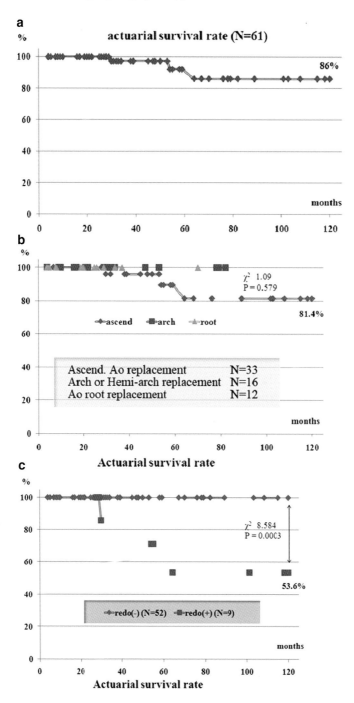

Fig. 1 Long-term results of emergency graft replacement for acute type A aortic dissection

surgery" strategy, in which root replacement and/or arch replacement were performed only when an intimal tear was present in the aortic segment(s).
- On the other hand, the minimal surgery strategy in the acute phase, as compared with more aggressive replacement option [2], is more likely to necessitate additional operation in the chronic phase, which caused significantly lower long-term survival rate as compared with the patients without redo surgery (See Fig.1c).

Of the 9 patients who needed redo surgery, 2 patients underwent Bentall operation because of relatively early dehiscence of the intima in the aortic root, probably as a result of inappropriate use of GRF glue [3,4]. And in 2 other patients who needed arch replacement, intimal tear was present in the aortic arch in the first operation. These patients had evolving myocardial ischemia necessitating additional CABG, and we confined the graft replacement to the ascending aorta in order to minimize surgical invasiveness. For these 4 cases (44.4% of our redo cases), additional aortic surgery might have been able to be avoided if (1) the rule of "resection and replacement of the segment having an intimal tear" had been strictly followed and (2) the application of formaldehyde in the GRF glue had been kept at the lowest necessary amount.

Figure 2 shows the excised aortic root wall in a patient during redo surgery. Tarnished portion shows degeneration of the wall due to formaldehyde. (Aortic wall was, as it were, "fixed" with formalin.)

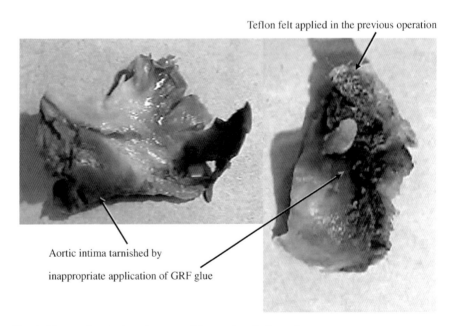

Fig. 2 Photos of excised aortic root wall in a patient during redo surgery

Conclusions

Emergency grafting for onset-phase acute type A aortic dissection could be performed with low operative mortality and satisfactory long-term survival rate. To improve the long-term results more, the rule of "resection and replacement of the segment having an intimal tear in the proximal aorta" should be strictly followed and (2) the formaldehyde used as a bridging agent of GRF glue be applied with the lowest necessary amount.

References

1. Ueda Y, Osada H, Osugi H (2007) Thoracic and cardiovascular surgery in Japan during 2005. Annual report by the Japanese Association for Thoracic Surgery. Gen Thorac Cardiovasc Surg 55:377–399
2. Watanuki H, Ogino H, Minatoya K, et al (2007) Is emergency total arch replacement with a modified elephant trunk technique justified for acute type A aortic dissection? Ann Thorac Surg 84:1585–91
3. Suzuki S, Imoto K, Uchida K, et al (2006) Aortic root necrosis after surgical treatment using gelatin-resorcinol-formaldehyde (GRF) glue in patients with acute type A aortic dissection. Ann Thorac Cardiovasc Surg 12:333–40
4. Kamada T, Nakajima T, Izumoto H, et al (2005) Late complications following surgery for type A acute aortic dissection using gelatin-resorcin-formaldehyde glue: report of two cases. Surg Today 35:996–9

Perioperative Risk Factors for Hospital Mortality in Patients with Acute Type A Aortic Dissection

Masashi Tanaka, Naoyuki Kimura, Hideo Adachi, Atsushi Yamaguchi, and Takashi Ino

Background: We investigated to determine risk factors for hospital mortality following surgery for acute type A aortic dissection (AAAD).

Method: Between January 1997 and December 2006, 243 consecutive patients with AAAD (127 men, 63 ± 11 years,) underwent emergent surgery at our hospital. Surgical procedures included hemiarch replacement (n = 204) and total or partial arch replacement (n = 31). Concomitant procedures included CABG (n = 17), aortic root replacement (n = 8), and aortic valve replacement (n = 3). Clinical data (30 variables) of these patients were analyzed retrospectively to determine independent risk factors for hospital mortality.

Results: Hospital mortality was 6.9% (17/243), and causes of hospital mortality included cardiac failure in 6, hemorrhage in 4, rupture of false lumen in 4, visceral ischemia in 2, and neurological deficits in 1 patient. Preoperative shock, preoperative intubation, prolonged operation time (> 6 hours), prolonged CPB time (> 4 hours) were revealed as risk factors by univariate analysis. Multivariate analysis indicated that preoperative shock ($p = 0.031$) and prolonged operation time ($p = 0.026$) as independent risk factors.

Conclusions: Preoperative shock and prolonged operation time (> 6 hours) were identified as independent risk factors for hospital mortality. Our findings may facilitate estimation of operative risk in individual patients.

M. Tanaka, N. Kimura, H. Adachi, A. Yamaguchi, and T. Ino
Department of Cardiovascular Surgery, Saitama Medical Center, Jichi Medical School, Saitama, Japan

M. Tanaka (✉)
Saitama Medical Center, Jichi Medical School, Saitama, Japan

Influence of Patent False Lumen on Secondary Dilation of the Distal Aorta Following Surgery for Acute Type A Aortic Dissection

Naoyuki Kimura, Masashi Tanaka, Hideo Adachi,
Atsushi Yamaguchi, and Takashi Ino

Background: The aim of this study was to assess the influence of residual patent false lumen on secondary dilation of the distal aorta following surgery of acute type A aortic dissection (AAAD).

Method: Between 1997 and 2006, 243 patients underwent emergency operation for AAAD. In-hospital mortality rate was 7.0 % (17/243). Of the discharged patients, 156 patients (69%) underwent at least 2 CT scans postopeatively at least 6 months interval (mean, 35 ± 24 months). These patients (mean age, 63 years) were divided into two groups according to the initial status of the false lumen; patent group (n = 100), and thrombosed group (n = 56). In each group, segment-specific aortic growth rate were calculated.

Results: At aortic arch (+1.7 vs. − 0.80 mm/y, p < .001), upper descending aorta (+1.6 vs. −0.41 mm/y, p = .005), and lower descending aorta (+0.89 vs −0.91 mm/y, p = .018), the average growth rate of patent group was significantly greater than thrombosed group. At abdominal aorta, there were no significant differences between the groups (+1.3 vs +0.80 mm/y, p = .46).

Conclusions: Residual patent false lumen influences postoperative enlargement of the distal aorta. Careful follow-up is important in patients with patent false lumen.

Penetrating Atherosclerotic Ulcer Causing Cardiac Tamponade – A Case Suggesting the Etiology of Intramural Hematoma

Nobuhiko Mukohara, Masato Yoshida, Satoshi Tobe, and Takashi Azami

We report a case of penetrating atherosclerotic causing cardiac tamponade and subadventitial hematoma. A 72-year-old man was transferred with sudden onset of chest pain and a subsequent collapse. A computed tomography scan showed a pericardial effusion and a low density shadow around the ascending aorta. An emergency operation was conducted with a diagnosis of intramural hematoma complicating cardiac tamponade.The patient underwent replacement of the ascending aorta. The specimen of the ascending aorta showed severe atherosclerosis and no intramural hematoma. Histological evaluation revealed a hemorrhage which connected a small intimal ulcer to the subadventitial hematoma. We think this case suggest the entry oriented etiology of intramural hematoma not rupture of a vasa vasorum.

N. Mukohara and M. Yoshida
Department of Cardiovascular Surgery, Hyogo Brain and Heart Center at Himeji, Japan

S. Tobe
Akashi Medical Center, Akashi, Japan

T. Azami
Yodogawa Christian Hospital, Osaka, Japan

Outcome of Patients with Acute Aortic Intramural Hematoma in the Extremely Early Stage

Hideyasu Kohshoh, Hideaki Yoshino, Hisashi Shimizu, Yasuhiro Ieizumi, Tatsuo Kikuchi, Takumi Inami, Wataru Nagai, Kenji Shida, Kenichi Sudo, and Yoshihiro Yamaguchi

Background: Natural history of aortic intramural hematoma (IMH) is still controversial. Previous reports on the prognosis of acute aortic dissection (AAD) have investigated the survival cases. The clinical courses of AAD during hyperacute phase before arrival to the hospital have yet to be clarified.

Methods: Among patients who were transfered our hospital in CPAOA, the prevalence of AAD with pericardial effusion was evaluated, as well as among AAD with cardiac tamponade, who were alive upon arrival during the same period.

Results: Among consecutive 1750 patients of CPAOA which underwent echocardiography and CT, 46 patients were diagnosed with Stanford type A AAD with massive pericardial effusion. Of 46 patients, 30 with a ring-shaped high-density lesion on the aortic wall in plain CT, which were diagnosed of IMH. Eighty-Three living patients were diagnosed of Type A [IMH: 39, PSL: 44]. Incidence of cardiac tamponade in the IMH was higher than that in the PSL [24/39 vs. 13/44, p = 0.003]. Among CPAOA with pericardial effusion and alive patients, incidence of cardiac tamponade in the IMH was higher than PSL [54/69 vs. 29/60, p<0.001].

Conclusion: Stanford type A IMH is frequently complicated with cardiac tamponade and causes a poor outcome in the extremely early stage.

Borderline Mesenteric Ischemia Caused by Acute Aortic Dissection

Borderline Mesenteric Ischemia in Aortic Dissection

Kazumasa Orihashi, Taijiro Sueda, Kenji Okada, and Katsuhiko Imai

Summary To make a diagnosis of mesenteric ischemia in acute aortic dissection, we have examined superior mesenteric artery (SMA) with transesophageal echocardiography (TEE) in addition to CT scan, and experienced borderline mesenteric ischemia, which is to be presented. The SMA was visualized with TEE by advancing the probe into the stomach and directing the transducer posteriorly. The TEE findings of SMA was correlated to the clinical course and CT findings in 28 cases with aortic dissection that extended to the abdominal aorta. Borderline mesenteric ischemia was found in four patients (14.3%). Preoperative CT showed patent and opaque SMA. However, TEE revealed narrowed true lumen in the proximal SMA or obstructed orifice of SMA by intimal flap. Two patients developed bowel necrosis and died. One patient underwent revascularization surgery. In another patient, obstruction of SMA orifice by intimal flap was released within 24 hours by spontaneous tear of flap and subsequent depressurization of false lumen. This patient had mild bloody stool and transient septic shock but they improved. There are cases with borderline mesenteric ischemia as well as those with totally necrotic intestine. TEE may provide additional information for assessing mesenteric ischemia in acute aortic dissection.

Keywords aortic dissection · mesenteric ischemia · transesophageal echocardiography · ultrasonography

---

K. Orihashi, T. Sueda, K. Okada, and K. Imai
Division of Cardiovascular Surgery, Hiroshima University Hospital

K. Orihashi (✉)
Division of Cardiovascular Surgery, Hiroshima University Hospital,
Kasumi 1-2-3, Minami-ku, Hiroshima, 734-8551 Japan
e-mail: orichan@hiroshima-u.ac.jp

Introduction

To make an early diagnosis of mesenteric ischemia, we have previously reported that transesophageal echocardiography (TEE) of the superior mesenteric artery (SMA) can be used to diagnose mesenteric ischemia [1]. Among the four types of aortic dissection, type C with a narrowed true lumen in the SMA compressed by an expanded false lumen and type D with an intimal flap obstructing the orifice of the SMA were considered to be at increased risk of mesenteric ischemia. In this report, we describe four cases of borderline mesenteric ischemia in types C and D aortic dissection.

Materials and Methods

We examined 28 consecutive cases with aortic dissection that extended to the abdominal aorta. The SMA was visualized with TEE by advancing the probe into the stomach and directing the transducer posteriorly [2]. After the celiac artery appeared, the SMA was visualized. The SMA was scanned in 0° and 90° to obtain both short- and long-axis views. The TEE findings on the SMA were correlated with the clinical course and CT findings.

Results

The results are listed in Table 1. We experienced four cases with borderline mesenteric ischemia. None of these patients had typical symptoms or apparent findings indicative of mesenteric ischemia. No patient had abdominal pain. Although acidosis was present, it was not specific for mesenteric ischemia. The SMA was patent based on the CT scan. The TEE finding was type C dissection in one patient

Table 1 Clinical appearances of four cases

case	1	2	3	4
pain	no	no	no	no
bowel sounds	±	±	±	good
acidosis	+	+	+	±
melena	± postop.	+ postop.	none	+ later
CT SMA	patent	patent	patent	occluded distal:patent
TEE type	B→C	D	D	D
Operation	Ao repair FL perfusion	Ao repair AMI	SMA bypass prev. CABG	none
prognosis	dead MOF	dead MOF	survived Ao repair	survived

SMA: superior mesenteric artery, FL: false lumen, AMI: acute myocardial infarction, CABG: coronary artery bypass grafting, MOF: multiple organ failure.

and type D in three patients. In case #1, the diagnosis based on TEE changed from type B to type C. Two of the four patients died.

Case #1 with type A dissection underwent ascending aorta repair. Femoral perfusion caused false lumen perfusion leading to cerebral malperfusion, and the arterial line was changed to the axillary artery. Despite the restoration of cerebral perfusion, acidosis remained after surgery. Although mesenteric ischemia was suspected from the TEE findings, surgery was not indicated because of multiple organ damage. The patient died two weeks later and the autopsy revealed: 1) dissection extending into SMA; 2) a narrowed true lumen in the SMA; and 3) diffuse necrosis of the intestine.

Case #2 had type A dissection (Marfan) with right coronary artery obstruction and underwent ascending aorta repair with coronary revascularization. The true lumen in the descending aorta was compressed by the expanded false lumen. Although the celiac artery and SMA were radio-opaque in the CT scan, intraoperative TEE showed a narrowed SMA orifice due to a displaced intimal flap. Because of myocardial ischemia, we placed priority on central repair. However, the base excess was <10 mEq/L and lactate reached 20.8 mmol/L during cardiopulmonary bypass. Although the laboratory data improved after surgery, she complained of abdominal pain with a paralytic intestine. Abdominal surgery was delayed due to sustained heart failure. Multiple organ failure progressed and she died on day 63 after surgery.

Case #3 had previous coronary revascularization seven months before and developed type A dissection. He complained of paresthesia bilaterally in his arms. CT showed that the true lumen in the abdominal aorta was narrowed, but the SMA was patent. The ultrasonic flow signal in the SMA was very weak, while it was apparent in the aorta that was more distant from the transducer than the SMA. Left iliac-SMA anastomosis and fenestration of the bilateral axillary artery were performed. Color and peristaltic movement of the intestine, and the acidosis improved after reperfusion of the SMA.

Case #4 had type B aortic dissection due to a traffic accident. CT showed that the true lumen was collapsed in the descending-to-abdominal aorta. The SMA was nearly occluded in the proximal portion but patent in the distal portion, perfused through collateral circulation from the colica media artery. She had no abdominal pain. Ultrasonography showed good bowel movement. The next day, the true lumen of the abdominal aorta as well as SMA expanded, because a detached flap at the orifice of the celiac artery functioned as a new site for blood entry. She had a small amount of blood in her stool on the first day and tarry stool for several days thereafter. She was discharged without significant sequelae.

Discussion

Mesenteric ischemia in aortic dissection is not always clinically apparent at the onset, but may later become significant. Early diagnosis and appropriate treatment without delay is essential for a good outcome. However, diagnosing mesenteric ischemia shortly after the onset of type A dissection is not always easy. Although CT is the first choice for initial assessment of the entire aorta, TEE and ultrasonography may provide additional information for assessing mesenteric ischemia in acute aortic dissection.

References

1. Orihashi K, Sueda T, Okada K, et al (2005) Perioperative diagnosis of mesenteric ischemia in acute aortic dissection by transesophageal echocardiography. Eur J Cardiothorac Surg 28:871–6
2. Orihashi K, Matsuura Y, Sueda T, et al (1998) Abdominal aorta and visceral arteries visualized with transesophageal echocardiography during operations on the aorta. J Thorac Cardiovasc Surg 115:945–7

Validity of Using Ghent Criteria for Japanese Population Suspected of Marfan Syndrome

Koichi Akutsu, Hiroko Morisaki, Takayuki Morisaki, Hitoshi Ogino,
Masashiro Higashi, Shingo Sakamoto, Tsuyoshi Yoshimuta,
Kazuya Okajima, Hiroshi Nonogi, and Satoshi Takeshita

Background: Diagnosis of Marfan syndrome (MFS) has been made based on Ghent criteria. However, there exist differences in habitus between Japanese and Western populations. We examined the validity to use Ghent criteria for Japanese populations suspected of MFS.

Methods: Seventy-four patients suspected of MFS were recruited. All patients received genetic analysis. Among 74 patients, 29 fulfilled Ghent criteria, and 25 of 29 showed mutations in the fibrillin-1 gene (13 men, 40 ± 10 yrs). Manifestation of these 25 patients with genetically proven MFS was evaluated according to Ghent criteria.

Results: Arm span to height ratio greater than 1.05 was observed in 13% (3/24), wrist and thumb sign in 72% (18/25), ectopia lentis in 39% (9/23), dilatation of the ascending aorta in 96% (23/24), mitral valve prolapse in 58% (14/24), striae atrophicae in 60% (12/20), and dural ectasia in 22% (5/23).

Conclusions: Among patients with genetically proven MFS, arm span to height ratio greater than 1.05, which is recognized as one of the most characteristic manifestations of MFS, was observed in less than 20% of the patients. Dural ectasia, which was reportedly observed in over 90% of MFS, was found in about 20%. Using Ghent criteria for the diagnosis of MFS in Japanese population may need further consideration.

K. Akutsu, S. Sakamoto, T. Yoshimuta, K. Okajima, H. Nonogi, and S. Takeshita
Department of Cardiovascular Medicine, National Cardiovascular Center, Suita, Japan

H. Morisaki and T. Morisaki
Department of Bioscience, National Cardiovascular Center, Suita, Japan

H. Ogino
Department of Cardiovascular Surgery, National Cardiovascular Center, Suita, Japan

M. Higashi
Department of Radiology, National Cardiovascular Center, Suita, Japan

Three Cases of Total Aortic Replacement for Marfan Syndrome

Eiichiro Inagaki, Sohei Hamanaka, Hisao Masaki, Masao Nakata, Atsushi Tabuchi, Yasuhiro Yunoki, Katsuhiko Shimizu, Yuji Hirami, Hitoshi Minami, Hiroshi Kubo, Takuro Yukawa, and Kazuo Tanemoto

Marfan syndrome is a connective tissue metabolic disorder which descends as autosomal dominant manner. Patients with Marfan syndrome suffer from various diseases such as aortic aneurysm or aortic dissection. We report three cases of total aortic replacement for Marfan syndrome.

Case 1: The first surgery was for the ruptured abdominal aortic aneurysm at his age of 21. This patient underwent surgeries three times by his age of 39.

Case 2: She underwent the first surgery for type IIIb aortic dissection when she was 50-year-old. Three surgeries were required for total aortic replacement by the *age of 63*.

Case 3: The first surgery was for type IIIb aortic dissection which had occurred when she was pregnant. Three surgeries were performed by her age of 32. Since patients with Marfan syndrome require multiple surgeries, the first operation should be planned considering the procedure of the next surgery. Elephant trunk or reversed elephant trunk are useful procedures for making the next surgery as easy as possible.

E. Inagaki, S. Hamanaka, H. Masaki, M. Nakata, A. Tabuchi, Y. Yunoki, K. Shimizu, Y. Hirami, H. Minami, H. Kubo, T. Yukawa, and K. Tanemoto
Division of Thoracic and Cardiovascular Surgery, Department of Surgery,
Kawasaki Medical School, Kurashiki, Japan

Aortic Operations in 150 Patients with Marfan Syndrome: Tokyo Experience

Takashi Azuma, Shigeyuki Aomi, Masayuki Miyagishima,
Hideyuki Tomioka, Satoshi Saito, Kenji Yamazaki, Akihiko Kawai,
and Hiromi Kurosawa

Background: Due to improved diagnostic and early surgical intervention, the life expectancy of patients with Marfan syndrome could be considerably improved. This study reviews the surgical outcome of patients who underwent aortic surgery in our institute.

Method: During a 28-year period, 155 patients underwent 228 operations on the aorta including 105 aortic root operation, 51 aortic arch operation, 26 descending thoracic aortic repairs, 30 thoracoabdominal aortic repairs, and 16 abdominal repairs.

Results: There were 5 operative deaths (3.2%) after the 228 operations. Survival after initial operation was 93.2%+/−2.0% at 1 year, 84.7%+/−3.0% at 5 years, and 82.9%+/−3.2% at 10 years. 52 (22.8%) patients underwent second operation in 5.2 years interval and 15 (6.5 %) underwent third operation 8.2 years interval. Re-operation free ratio was 95.2%+/−1.6% at 1 year, 78.3%+/−3.6% at 5 years, and 70.2%+/−4.4% at 10 years. Re-operation include 13 in aortic root, 8 in aortic arch, 8 in descending thoracic aorta, 12 in thoracoabdominal aorta, and 9 in abdominal aorta. Total aortic replacement was achieved in 7 cases in 11.7+/−4.5 years.

Conclusion: Early and long term results of aortic surgery in Japanese Marfan patient were excellent. Multiple staged procedure with careful observation could be attributed to this favorable outcome.

T. Azuma, S. Aomi, M. Miyagishima, H. Tomioka, S. Saito, K. Yamazaki,
A. Kawai, and H. Kurosawa
Department of Cardiovascular Surgery, Tokyo Women's Medical University, Tokyo, Japan

Poster Session 2
Extensive Surgery, Root, Arch and Therocoabdomonal Aorta

Surgery for Extensive Thoracic Aortic Aneurysm

Hiroshi Munakata, Kenji Okada, Akiko Tanaka, Masamichi Matsumori, Mitsuru Asano, Yoshihisa Morimoto, and Yutaka Okita

Summary

Objective: Surgical strategy for extensive thoracic aortic aneurysms (ETAA) was investigated.

Methods: Forty-three consecutive patients underwent the repair of ETAA from 1999 to 2007. There were 17 patients in one stage group (63.2 ± 11.3y), while 21 patients in staged repair group (60.3 ± 16.6y). All patients in one stage group, underwent the ascending aorta and aortic arch replacement in combined with various extensions of descending aortic replacement (proximal 5, middle 8, total descending 1, or thoracoabdominal aorta 3). In staged repair group, second-stage repair were performed (Surgery: 14, Stent graft 7) after the first-stage graft replacement (total arch replacement (TAR) 7, TAR + aortic root replacement (ARR) 7, TAR + Coronary artery bypass grafting ± ARR 7).

Results: Hospital mortality was 12.0% (2/17) in one stage repair and 9.0% (4/21) in staged repair. There was no significant difference in morbidity, late mortality and freedom from vascular related death between two groups.

Conclusion: Surgical outcome for ETTA was satisfactory in both one stage and staged repair groups. One stage surgery could be first choice in carefully selected patients.

Keywords Extensive thoracic aortic aneurysm · One stage repair · Staged repair · Surgical results

---

H. Munakata, K. Okada, A. Tanaka, M. Matsumori, M. Asano, Y. Morimoto, and Y. Okita
Division of Cardiovascular Surgery, Kobe University Graduate School of Medicine

Y. Okita (✉)
Kobe University Hospital, Department of Cardiovascular, Thoracic, and Pediatric Surgery,
7-5-2, Kusunoki-cho, Chuo-ku, Kobe, Japan
e-mail: yokita@med.kobe-u.ac.jp

Introduction

Surgical repair of extensive thoracic aortic aneurysms (ETAA) remains challenging because of its high mortality and morbidity. Surgical modes of one stage [1–4] or staged repair [5–8] was determined based on the aneurysmal anatomy and comorbidity, however the patients' selection was still controversial. The purpose of the present study was to analyze surgical outcome for the ETAA comparing with these two strategies.

Material and Methods

Within recent 8 years, 43 consecutive patients underwent the repair of ETAA and 38 patients were included in this study. The selection of surgery has shown in Fig. 1. With regard to patient's profile and pre-operative comorbidity, chronic aortic dissection was the principal indication for one stage repair. There was significant difference only in the incident of dissection between one stage and staged repair (acute dissection: 3 vs 0, p=0.041, chronic dissection: 14 vs. 7, p=0.003, rupture: 2 vs 0, p=0.08, Emergency: 4 vs 2, p=0.21, COPD: 1 vs 3, p=0.20, coronary disease: 2 vs 7, p=0.14, renal dysfunction: 6 vs 6 p=0.57, cerebrovascular disease: 2 vs 6, p=0.18). With regard to distal extension of procedures, staged repair group involved more extensive compared with one stage group. (Table 1)

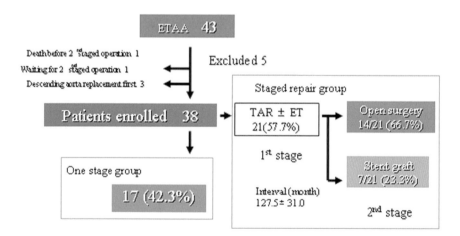

Fig. 1 Our surgical strategy. Forty-three consecutive patients underwent the repair of ETAA from 1999 to 2007, 5 patients were excluded. Surgical modes were selected based on the aneurysmal anatomy and patients comorbidity. ETAA: Extensive thorasic aortic aneurysm TAR: Total arch replacement ET: Elephant trunk

Table 1 One stage repair

Previous procedures	No. of patients (%)
Hemiarch replacement	11 (65)
Bentall operation	1 (6)
Stent graft (TEVER)	1 (6)
No previous operation	4 (23)
Extent of descending thoracic aortic lesion	
Proximal	5 (29)
Middle	8 (47)
Distal	1 (6)
Thoracoabdominal aorta	3 (17)

Staged repair

Stage 1 surgery	No. of patients (%)
Total arch replacement (TAR)	7 (33)
TAR+Aortic root replacement (ARR)	7 (33)
TAR+Coronary artery bypass+ARR	7 (33)
Extent of descending thoracic aortic lesion	
Proximal	4 (19)
Middle	4 (19)
Distal	3 (17)
Thoracoabdominal aorta	10 (47)
2nd stage method	
Surgery	14 (67)
Descending aortic replacement	4 (19)
Thoracoabdominal aortic replacement	8 (38)
Total arch replacement	2 (9)
Stent graft (TEVAR)	7 (33)

Statistical Analysis

Comparisons between one stage or staged repair were analyzed using the χ^2 test and Student's t test. Survival in each group was analyzed with the Kaplan-Meier method and log-rank test.

Results

Hospital mortality was 12.0% (2/17: LOS 1, MOF 1) in one stage repair, while 9.0% (4/21: MOF 2, Pneumonia 1, graft infection 1) (p=0.72) in staged repair. There were no significant difference in morbidity between two groups (paraplegia: 0 vs 3, p=0.11, pulmonary complication: 2 vs 1, p=0.34, Transient neuralgic dysfunction: 2 vs 0, p=0.1, renal dialysis: 0 vs 0, heart failure: 0 vs 1, p=0.38).

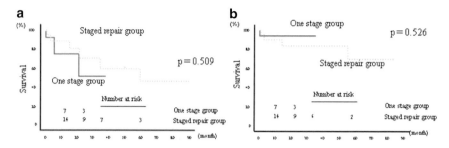

Fig. 2 (a) Long-term survival. Follow-up years; one staged repair group: 1.0 ± 0.85 years, staged repair group: 2.4 ± 2.3 years. (b) Freedom from vascular related death

Late mortality was 6.6% (1/15: MOF) in one stage repair and 17.6% (3/17: stent graft migration 1, unknown 1, respiratory failure 1) in staged repair. Mortality at one year was 21% in one stage group and 12% in staged group and mortality at 3-year was 40% and 34% respectively. Freedom from vascular related death at one year was 6% in one stage group and 10% in staged group and 3-year was 10% and 16%, which showed no significant difference (Fig. 2).

Discussion

The surgical treatment for ETAA that involves the ascending, arch, and descending aortic segments remains challenging because of substantial morbidity and mortality. There have been many reports describing surgical repair of ETAA by one stage [1–4] or staged repair [5–8], however, the optimal surgical strategy for ETAA remains unclear.

Some patients also require concomitant treatment of coronary artery or heart valve disease, staged repair is likely to be performed to gain access to all parts of the thoracic aorta and cardiac structures. This, however, exposes the patients to the risk of two major procedures. On the other hand, the one stage repair enables to avoid possible ruptures and aortic event during the interval. In our series, there was one patient whose residual aneurysm ruptured before second staged repair.

Our experience demonstrated that one staged repair has no additional risk of long-tem mortality and vascular related death, furthermore, there was no significant difference in morbidity. Therefore, we believe one stage repair could be applicable as long as patient's selection was carefully done.

Endovascular stenting of the descending aorta into the previous elephant trunk have been reported previously. The procedure potentially allowed the surgeon to avoid a second complex open procedure; however, the indication is limited to patients who meet certain anatomic criteria [8].

Conclusion

Our surgical outcome for the repair of extensive thoracic aneurysm was acceptable in both one stage and staged repairs. We believe one stage repair could be applicable for ETAA in selected patient's.

References

1. Nicholas TK, Michael CM, Paolo Masetti, et al (2007) Optimization of Aortic Arch Replacement With a One-Stage Approach. Ann Thorac Surg 83:S811–S814
2. Hu XP, Chang Q, Zhu JM, et al (2006) One-Stage Total or Subtotal Aortic Replacement. Ann Thorac Surg 82:542–546
3. Massimo CG, Perna AM, Cruz Quadron EA,et al (1997) Extended and total simultaneous aortic replacement: latest technical modifications and improved results with thirty-four patients. J Card Surg 12:261-9
4. Doss M, Woehleke T, Wood JP, et al (2003) The clamshell approach for the treatment of extensive thoracic aortic disease. J Thorac Cardiovasc Surg 126:814-7
5. Safi HJ, Miller CC 3rd, Estrera AL, et al (2007) Optimization of Aortic Arch Replacement: Two-Stage Approach. Ann Thorac Surg 83:S815–S818
6. LeMaire SA, Carter SA, Coselli JS (2006) The elephant trunk technique for staged repair of complex aneurysms of the entire thoracic aorta. Ann Thorac Surg 81:1561-9
7. Borst HG, Walterbusch G, Schaps D, et al (1983) Extensive aortic replacement using "elephant trunk" prosthesis, Thorac Cardiovasc Surg 31:37–40
8. Azizzadeh A, Estrera AL, Porat EE, et al (2006) The hybrid elephant trunk procedure: A single stage repair of an ascending, arch, and descending thoracic aortic aneurysm. J Vasc Surg 44:404-7

Surgical Strategy in Aortic Lesion for Marfan Syndrome

Akiko Tanaka, Kenji Okada, Hiroshi Munakata, Masamichi Matsumori, and Yutaka Okita

Objectives: The purpose of this study was to investigate our current surgical strategy in treating aortic disease in Marfan syndrome.

Methods: Thirty-one patients with Marfan syndrome underwent aortic repair in past eight years. Our current strategy is to apply aortic root replacement with David valve-sparing procedure in patients with annuloaortic ectasia (AAE) whose root diameter exceeds 40 mm, total arch replacement with elephant trunk installation (TAR+ET) in addition to ascending or root replacement to type A dissection (AD-A), and one-stage thoracoabdominal aortic replacement to type B dissection (AD-B). In 28 patients with AAE, 19 David's reimplantation technique and 8 Bentall's operation were performed. In 6 AD-A patients, 3 Bentall operation and 1 one reimplantation operation were performed and 5 concomitant TAR+ETs were applied in 5 cases. In 12 AD-B patients, one-stage repair was performed in 7 cases.

Results: There was no mortality, paraplegia or stroke in this series. Subsequent operations were required in 16 patients for newly developed AD-B or AAE, enlargement of the residual dissection, and failure of valve-sparing technique estimated by the Kaplan-Meier method was 86.7% at 1 year and 54.4% in 5 years.

Conclusions: Our surgical results for aortic patients with Marfan was satisfactory.

Keywords Marfan syndrome · annuloaortic ectasia · dissection · surgical strategy · reimplantation

---

A. Tanaka, K. Okada, H. Munakata, M. Matsumori, and Y. Okita
Division of Cardiovascular Surgery, Department of Surgery,
Kobe University Graduate School of Medicine

A. Tanaka (✉)
Division of Cardiovascular Surgery, Department of Surgery,
Kobe University Graduate School of Medicine
7-5-2 Kusunoki-cho, Chuo-ku, Kobe 650-0017, Japan
e-mail: akikotanaka623@yahoo.co.jp

Introduction: The vast majority of Marfan patients eventually develop cardiovascular complications because of their genetic disorders, and the cardiovascular events determine their prognosis. The purpose of this study was to investigate our current surgical strategy in treating aortic disease in patients with Marfan syndrome.

Methods: From April 1999 to April 2007, 31 Marfan syndrome patients, with mean age of 38.6±13.6 years at first operation, were referred to our institute for surgical intervention in aortic lesions. There were 12 males. Our current strategy for aortic disease in Marfan syndrome is to apply aortic root replacement with valve-sparing operation in patients with annuloaortic ectasia (AAE) whose root diameter exceeds 40 mm, total arch replacement with elephant trunk installation (TAR+ET) in addition to ascending or root replacement to type A dissection (AD-A), and one-stage thoracoabdominal aortic replacement to type B dissection (AD-B) whose aortic diameter exceeds 50 mm.

Total of 58 operations was performed, including 19 procedures previously performed at other institutions. The indications and procedures are listed in Table 1. The most common surgery was aortic root replacement accounting for 90.3% (28 of 31)

Table 1 Operative indications and procedures performed

Indications	Procedures	1st	2nd	3rd	4th	5th
AAE and/or AR without dissection						
	David	13	3			
	Bentall	4	1			
	root replacement		1			
	David + TAR + ET	1			1	
AD-A						
	David + TAR + ET		1			
	Bentall	1				
	Bentall + TAR + ET	2				
	TAR+ET	2	1			
	descending Ao		1			
	TAAA			1		
AD-B						
	TAAA	2	6	3	1	
	Descending Ao	3	1			
	AAA			2		
Valves						
	MVP	1				
	MVR	1				1
	AVR	1	2	1		

AAE: annuloaortic ectasia, AR: aortic regurgitation, AD-A: type A dissection, AD-B: type B dissection, TAR: total arch replacement, ET: total arch replacement and elephant trunk installation, Descending Ao: descending aorta grafting, TAAA: thoracoabdominal aortic aneurysm grafting, AAA: abdominal aortic aneurysm grafting, MVP: mitral valve plasty, MVR: mitral valve replacement, AVR: aortic valve replacement.

of the entity. Among them, Bentall's operation, David's type valve-sparing technique, and root replacement were performed in 8, 19, and 1 patients respectively.

Follow up was 100% complete either with periodical follow up at our institute or telephone interview and the mean follow up of 82.7±60.7 months which was calculated from the date of the first operation.

Results: Preoperative diameter of Valsalva sinus in Bentall's operation group was 63.0±4.1 mm whereas in reimplantation group was 47.8±6.8 mm. Preoperative AR grade in Bentall's operation group was 3.3±0.6°/ 4°while in reimplantation group was 2.0±1.2°/4°. Postoperative AR grade in the reimplantation group improved to 0.8±0.8°/4°.

There was no overall mortality. Major morbidity was seen in 7 cases (2 re-exploration for bleeding, 1 complete atrioventricular, 1 graft branch occlusion treated with interventional radiology, 1 temporary dysphasia, and 1 graft infection after thoracoabdomial aorta replacement, in which closed continuous irrigation was performed for 5 months and subsequent re-mitral valve replacement was applied for prosthetic valve infection (PVE)). There was no stroke, paraplegia or paraparesis seen in all procedures. Major adverse cardiac and aortic events (MACAE) were seen in 17 patients (57.8%), and all events were reoperation or subsequent surgeries with total of 27 procedures. The surgical indications for those were newly developed lesions (AD-A, ADB or AAE) in 14 cases, enlargement of the residual dissection in 9 cases, failure after the valve-sparing technique in 3 cases (two cases were initially operated in other centers), and PVE in 1 case. The mean interval between the first and the second operation was 49.5±52.7 months. Overall freedom from MACAE estimated by the Kaplan-Meier method was 86.7% at 1 year and 54.4% in 5 years.

Discussion: Our result in reimplantation was comparable with that of Bentall operation [1, 2]. Considering the low risk thromboembolic or bleeding events, Marfan patients may benefit more from the valve-sparing procedures.

Natural history of Marfan revealed that earlier intervention before aortic rupture of dissection prolonged the prognosis of these patients [3, 4].

Marfan patients often require downstream aortic surgery when they were operated for dissection [4–7]. In our series, there were 5 of 6 AD-A patients (including 1 patient after graft replacement of descending aorta for AD-B) had transverse aortic arch replaced at the initial operation for AD-A and the rest of 1 patient also eventually required TAR+ET as a result of rapid enlargement in the dissected arch. We also performed 10 one-stage TAAR and the staged TAAR was required in 4 cases of 18 dissected thoracoabdominal aorta. We strongly recommend TAR + ET for AD-A in Marfan patient. Also considering the age and low risk of paraplegia in aortic surgery in Marfan's syndrome [8] and to avoid re-thoracotomy, one-stage TAAR is preferable.

Conclusion: Mid-term results of reimplantation technique in Marfan syndrome was satisfactory and extensive aortic reconstruction can be performed with low morbidity and mortality in this entity. Considering the vast majority of indivisuals with Marfan are in young age, our strategy can be beneficial to them in regard to anticoagulant free life and reducing number of additional or repetitive surgery.

References

1. Karck M, Kallenbach K, Hagi C, et al (2004) Aortic Root Surgery in Marfan Syndrome. J Thorac Cardiovasc Surg 127:391–8
2. Oliveira NC, David TE, Ivanov J, et al (2003) Results of Aortic Aneurysm in Patients with Marfan syndrome. J Thorac Cardiovasc Surg 125:789–96
3. Gott WL, Greeene PS, Alejp DE, et al (1999) Replacement of the Aortic Root in Patients with Marfan's syndrome. N Engl J Med 340:1307–13
4. Milewicz D, Dietz HC, Miller DC (2005) Treatment of Aortic Disease in Patients with Marfan Syndrome. Circulation 111:150–7
5. Bachet J, Larrazet F, Goudot B, et al (2007) When Should the Aortic Arch Be Replaced in Marfan Patients? Ann Thorac Surg 83:S774–9
6. Tagusari O, Ogino H, Kobayashi J (2004) Should the Transverse Aortic Arch Be Replaced Simultaneously with Aortic Root Replacement for Annuloaortic Ectasia in Marfan Syndrome? J Thorac Cardiovasc Surg 127:1373–80
7. Finkbohner R, Johnston D, Crawford ES, et al (1995) Long-Term Survival and Complications After Aortic Aneurysm Repair. Circulation 91:728–3
8. Coselli JS, LeMaire SA, Buker Suat (1995) Marfan Syndrome: The Variability and Outcome of Operative Management. J Vasc Surg 21:432–43

One-stage Repair of Total Descending Aorta for Extended Pathologies

Tetsuro Morota, Shinichi Takamoto, Tetsufumi Yamamoto, Kan Nawata, and Mitsuhiro Kawata

Summary

Objectives: One of the potential solutions for embolic events in aortic surgery is to perform aggressive replacement for extended pathologies. The aim of this review was to assess outcomes for aggressive one-stage repair of total descending aorta.

Methods: Consecutive procedures, replacing the descending aorta at least from the distal arch to diaphragmatic crus, from March 2000 to May 2007 were reviewed. Our strategy consists of: 1; anterolateral thoracotomy through *single* 5th intercostal space with costal arch division, 2; "arch first" under deep hypothermic circulatory arrest with retrograde cerebral circulation, 3; open proximal anastomosis, 4; segmental clamping, 5; carbon dioxide insufflation.

Results: There were 36 patients, 28 men and 8 women, with a mean age of 62 yr, ranging 28–77. The type of aneurysm was dissection in 18, true aneurysm in 15, and combined lesion in 3. Four of them were emergent cases for symptomatic aneurysms. More extended replacement to the arch vessels was applied in 15 and to the abdominal vessels in 5. No hospital death, but serious stroke in 2 and delayed paraparesis in 1 occurred.

Conclusion: One-stage repair of total descending aorta provided excellent early results, prohibiting embolic events originated in extended pathologies.

Keywords aortic aneurysm · thoracotomy · circulatory arrest · retrograde cerebral perfusion · paraplegia

---

T. Morota, S. Takamoto, T. Yamamoto, K. Nawata, and M. Kawata
Department of Cardiothoracic Surgery, The University of Tokyo

T. Morota (✉)
Department of Cardiothoracic Surgery, The University of Tokyo
Hongo 7-3-1, Bunkyo-ku, Tokyo 113-8655, Japan
e-mail: morotat@hotmail.co.jp

Introduction

There has been significant increase in number of patients who undergo thoracic aortic surgery in the past decade. Among them, one of the most common and serious perioperative complications is embolic events, such as stroke, renal dysfunction, or mesenteric ischemia, since vast majority of the patients have diffuse, extended atherosclerosis in the descending thoracic aorta. Clamping the diseased aorta or leaving atheromatous lesion results in arterial embolism.

A possible solution to avoid embolic events is to perform extensive replacement of the total descending thoracic aorta, although the surgical invasiveness could be higher.

Materials and Methods

From March 2000 to May 2007, 36 patients, 28 men and 8 women, with a mean age of 62 yr, ranging 28–79, underwent one-stage repair of total descending aorta for extended pathologies. The term "one-stage repair of total descending aorta" was defined as "to replace at least distal arch to Th10 level descending aorta as a single procedure". The type of aneurysm was dissection in 18 patients, true aneurysm in 15, and combined lesion in 3. There were 9 patients with shaggy aorta and 1 patient with porcelain aorta. Four of them were emergent cases for symptomatic aneurysms. The concomitant procedures were described in Table 1.

Surgical Procedure

Anterolateral thoracotomy was carried out through single 5th intercostal space with costal arch division to obtain an optimal surgical view of the entire descending aorta. The arch aorta was reconstructed with so called "arch first technique" under deep hypothermic circulatory arrest and retrograde cerebral circulation [1] to minimize brain damage. For the purpose of spinal cord protection, "segmental clamping" was used whenever possible, and the body temperature was kept at moderate hypothermia until reperfusion of the intercostal arteries. During the procedure, carbon dioxide insufflation into the surgical field was used to reduce air embolisms.

Results

The operation data were demonstrated in Table 2. There was no operative or hospital mortality. Major stroke, with significant new lesion on brain CT, occurred in 2 patients and transient neurological deficit without significant new lesion occurred

Table 1 Concomitant procedures

	Number of cases
CABG	9
Arch replacement	15
Total arch	13
LSA	2
Visceral brances	5
CA	3
CA+SMA	1
CA+SMA+RAs	1
Intercostal arteries	25

CABG, coronary artery bypass grafting; LSA, left subclavian artery; CA, celiac artery; SMA, superior mesenteric artery; RAs, renal arteries.

Table 2 Operation data (in minutes)

	Mean	S.D.	Minimum	Maximum
Operation time	561	119	320	775
Pump run	299	67	177	408
RCC	51	14	25	83
Lower body CA	53	28	0	113

RCC, retrograde cerebral circulation; CA, circulatory arrest.

Table 3 Early surgical results

Hospital mortality	0
Morbidity	
Major stroke	2
Transient neurological deficit	4
Spinal cord injury (delayed parapare	1
respiratory failure	0
Renal dysfunction (Cr > 2.0)	11
Liver dysfunction (GOT and/or GPT > 100)	14
Hospitalization (mean ± SD)	32 ± 9 days

in 4 patients. One patient developed delayed paraparesis on the third postoperative day. There were no serious respiratory complications except one in a patient who required tracheotomy for prolonged consciousness disturbance after major stroke. Renal and liver function were maintained well although nearly one-third of the patients developed temporary dysfunction that was recovered within a couple of weeks. The early results were summarized in Table 3. After mean follow-up of 49 months, late death occurred in 5 patients; heart failure in 3, aspiration pneumonia in 1, rupture of infrarenal abdominal aorta in 1. No patients required re-thoracotomy so far.

Discussion

One-stage repair of total descending aorta eliminated the risk of atheromatous embolism. Although 2 patients were complicated with major stroke, all the patients in this series had extremely high risk for atheromatous embolism in manipulating the aorta, setting up cardiopulmonary bypass, and clamping the aorta. It was true that this procedure entailed significant longer time of operation and pump run, the patients tolerated well. For distal aortic anastomosis, lower half body circulatory arrest was employed to make open anastomosis in most of the patients, however, moderate hypothermia protected the visceral organs and minimized kidney and liver damage. As for visualization of the entire thoracic aorta, costal arch division gave us very good surgical field (Fig. 1a, b), from the ascending aorta to the lower descending aorta, even to the abdominal aorta when an extensive incision was made to open the retroperitoneal space. In spite of extended dissection of the aorta, no bleeding tendency was observed and no re-thoracotomy for bleeding was made.

As a tip in the wide opening of the thorax, we consider that the 4th intercostal should be cut posteriorly to the rib angle, close to the vertebra, from the thoracic cavity, without longer skin incision to the back. The latissimus dorsi muscle was preserved completely, and the serratus muscle was just divided in parallel with the muscle fibers. Then the respiratory muscles were preserved well and postoperative respiratory function was also maintained. On the other hand, this approach seemed to be technically difficult in certain patients with obesity, respiratory dysfunction, or heart dysfunction. And the longer operation time might risk in elderly patients.

It was speculated that the cause of 2 major strokes in this series was atheromatous embolism due to retrograde perfusion from the femoral artery. The pump perfusion line should be placed on the ascending aorta or the axillary artery [2], when there was serious atheromatous change in the abdominal aorta or iliac arteries.

Conclusion

One-stage repair of total descending aorta would be a justified procedure with acceptable surgical results in patients with extended aortic pathologies such as mega-aorta or chronic type B aortic dissection.

One-stage Repair of Total Descending Aorta

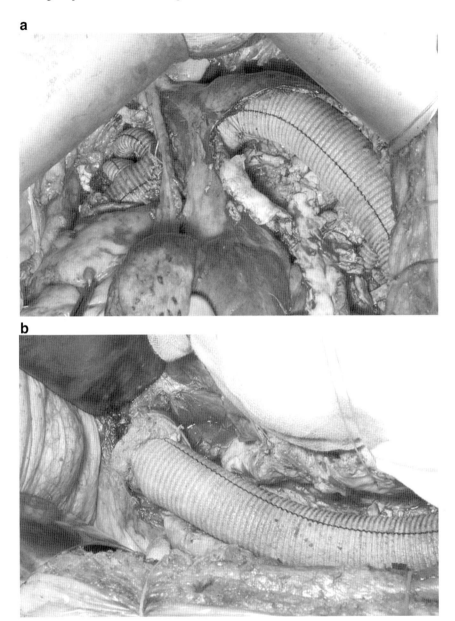

Fig. 1 Surgical view of "one-stage repair of total descending aorta". (**a**) The transverse arch to proximal descending aorta. White arrow: arch vessels. (**b**) The distal descending aorta. The anastomosis was made at Th11 level

References

1. Takamoto S, Okita Y, Ando M, et al (1994) Retrograde cerebral circulation for distal aortic arch surgery through a left thoracotomy. J Card Surg 9:576–583
2. Neri E, Massetti M, Vapannini G, et al (1999) Axillary artery cannulation in type A aortic dissection operations. J Thorac Cardiovasc Surg 118:324–329

Surgical Results of Descending Thoracic and Thoracoabdominal Aortic Aneurysm Repair Using deep Hypothermic Circulatory Arrest

Kazuhiro Naito, Masashi Tanaka, Hideo Adachi,
Atsushi Yamaguchi, and Takashi Ino

Background: To avoid thromboembolism and aortic wall injury of the clamp site, open proximal and/or distal anastomosis technique with deep hypothermic circulatory arrest (DHCA) has been positively applied for complex descending thoracic and thoracoabdominal aortic aneurysm repair in our institution. We examined early surgical results of 161 patients underwent descending thoracic and thoracoabdominal aortic aneurysm repair applying this technique.

Methods: Since October 1992, 161 (121 men, age 62.3 ± 13.3 years) of 239 patients underwent descending thoracic and thoracoabdominal aortic aneurysm repair applied DHCA (67.4 %). The etiology of aneurysm included degenerative (n=94), dissection (n=53), trauma (n=9), and others (n=4). Emergent surgery was performed in 41 patients (25.5 %).

Results: Replacement of descending thoracic aorta was performed in 138 and thoracoabdominal aorta in 23 patients. Open anastmosis technique was performed in proximal: 131, in distal: 131, and in both: 80. Hospital mortality was 8.1% (13/161) and causes of death were as follows; cardiac failure: 4, hemorrhage: 4, visceral ischemia: 3, sepsis: 2, pneumonia: 1. Postoperative complications included cerebral infarction: 11, acute renal failure: 8, paraplegia: 3.

Conclusions: Our surgical strategy for descending thoracic and thoracoabdominal aortic aneurysm repair seems to be pertinent with acceptable in-hospital results.

K. Naito, M. Tanaka, H. Adachi, A. Yamaguchi, and T. Ino
Department of Cardiothoracic Surgery, Jichi Medical School Saitama Medical Center, Saitama, Japan

Simultaneous Surgery for Thoracic Aortic Aneurysm with Coronary Artery Disease

Akihito Matsushita, Tatsuhiko Komiya, Nobushige Tamura, Genichi Sakaguchi, Taira Kobayashi, Tomokuni Furukawa, Gengo Sunagawa, and Takashi Murashita

Summary

Objective: We describe our strategy and the outcomes of simultaneous coronary artery bypass grafting (CABG) during surgery for thoracic aortic aneurysms in patients with coronary artery disease.

Patients and Methods: We enrolled 34 consecutive patients (age: 70.6 ± 10.9 years) who underwent simultaneous elective surgeries between June 2000 and June 2007. The aorta was replaced under cardiopulmonary bypass with moderate or profound hypothermia. We performed CABG while waiting for, and/or during recovery from hypothermia. The mean number of anastomoses was 1.8 ± 0.9, and the complete revascularization rate was 88.2%.

Results: One patient underwent postoperative percutaneous coronary intervention (PCI) for an occluded left internal thoracic artery. Three patients who underwent PCI and 1 who underwent pacemaker implantation because of SSS were defined as having late cardiac events. There were no in-hospital deaths, but 4 late deaths occurred due to non-cardiac problems (mean follow-up: 28.6 ± 22.2 months). The 3-year survival and cardiac-related event-free rates were 90.6% and 83.0%, respectively.

Conclusions: The early and late outcomes of simultaneous surgery for thoracic aortic aneurysm with coronary artery disease were satisfactory.

Keywords simultaneous surgery · thoracic aortic aneurysm · coronary artery disease · CABG · aortic replacement

---

A. Matsushita, T. Komiya, N. Tamura, G. Sakaguchi, T. Kobayashi, T. Furukawa, G. Sunagawa, and T. Murashita
Department of Cardiovascular Surgery, Kurashiki Central Hospital

A. Matsushita (✉)
Department of Cardiovascular Surgery, Kurashiki Central Hospital
1-1-1 Miwa, Kurashiki, Okayama 710-8602, Japan
e-mail: am8533@kchnet.or.jp

Introduction

When coronary artery disease coexists with thoracic aortic aneurysm (TAA), we perform simultaneous coronary artery bypass grafting (CABG) and surgery for the TAA. The incidence of this combination of disease ranges from 16 to 30% [1]. This means that coronary artery disease should be detected preoperatively and adequately managed in patients with TAA. We routinely perform CAG in patients with TAA with the objective of complete revascularization.

Some systematic investigations of simultaneous surgery have uncovered an unsatisfactory postoperative mortality rate between 12.5 and 27% [1–3]. We retrospectively analyzed patients who underwent simultaneous surgeries.

Patients and Methods

From June 2000 to June 2007, we applied elective TAA to 34 patients with coronary artery disease. Aortic replacement and CABG were performed under cardiopulmonary bypass (CPB). Table 1 summarizes the clinical characteristics of the study population. The clinical diagnoses of the patients were as follows: true aneurysm of the thoracic aorta, 30; annuloaortic ectasia, 3; true aneurysm of

Table 1 Characteristics of Patients

Number of patients	34
Mean age (years)	70.6 ± 10.9
Gender (Male/Female)	19/15
Left Ventricular Ejection Fraction	60.4 ± 11.1%
Hypertension	26/34 (76.4%)
Hyperlipidemia	13/34 (38.2%)
Diabetes mellitus (medication or insulin therapy)	2/34 (5.9%)
Hemodialysis	1/34 (2.9%)
Clinical diagnosis	Thoracic aortic aneurysm 30
	Annuloaortic ectasia 3
	Thoracoabdominal aneurysm 1
Coronary artery disease	Angina pectoris 29
	Old myocardial infarction 5
Operation: Aortic replacement + CABG	Replacement place of aorta
	Ascending aorta and aortic arch 14
	Ascending aorta 9
	Ascending aorta + hemi-aortic arch 4
	Aortic arch and descending aorta 4
	Aortic arch 2
	Thoracoabdominal aorta 1

*Six patients underwent aortic valve replacement, 2 underwent mitral valve plasty, and 2 underwent pulmonary vein isolation concomitantly.

the thoracoabdominal aorta, 1. Coronary artery diseases consisted of 29 angina pectoris and 5 old myocardial infarction. Six patients underwent concomitant aortic valve replacement because of aortic valve regurgitation. Various operations were performed in these patients (Table 1).

During ascending and/or aortic arch surgery was performed via a median sternotomy using CPB. An arterial cannula was inserted into the ascending aorta, and venous drainage was achieved via right atrial or bicaval cannulation. The bladder temperature was lowered to 20~28°C. Distal anastomoses of the graft-coronary artery were performed during core cooling. Cardioplegic solution was intermittently infused through an aortic root cannula and free grafts that were anastomosed to the coronary artery. The aorta was replaced under antegrade selective cerebral perfusion (SCP). Distal anastomosis was performed using the open distal and "turn-up" suture technique [4]. Distal body perfusion was reestablished through the branched graft, which was unclamped after reconstruction of the left subclavian artery and the proximal anastomosis was finished. The other arch branches were reconstructed and proximal anastomoses of the free grafts were completed during rewarming.

Results

The mean number of anastomosed coronary arteries was 1.8 ± 0.9 vessels per patient, and the complete revascularization rate was 88.2%. We used 24 left internal thoracic arteries (LITA), 20 saphenous vein grafts (SVG), 2 right internal thoracic arteries (RITA), 2 gastroepiploic arteries (GEA) and 2 radial arteries (RA). Thirteen SVGs and 2 RAs were anastomosed to the artificial graft, and the other free grafts were anastomosed to the ascending aorta. All patients underwent postoperative coronary angiography (CAG) about one week after surgery, and 48 patent and 2 occluded bypass grafts, indicated a graft patency rate of 96.0%. One patient underwent postoperative percutaneous coronary intervention (PCI). Table 2 shows that the postoperative patency rates of these grafts and of those in patients who underwent isolated CABG at our hospital from 1999 to 2006 did not significantly differ.

No morbidity was associated with TAA repair. Early postoperative morbidity comprised cerebral infarction, 1; pneumonia, 3 and paroxysmal atrial fibrillation, 8.

Table 2 Postoperative patency rates of CABG grafts

	Postoperative graft patency rate		
	Study group	Isolated CABG group 1999 ~ 2006	P value
LITA	95.8% (23/24)	97.4% (188/193)	P = 0.83
RITA	50.0% (1/2)	96.4% (27/28)	P = 0.13
RA	100% (2/2)	100% (118/118)	P = 1.00
SVG	100% (20/20)	93.9% (78/83)	P = 0.58
GEA	100% (2/2)	100% (49/49)	P = 1.00

*Patients underwent CAG about 1 week after operation.

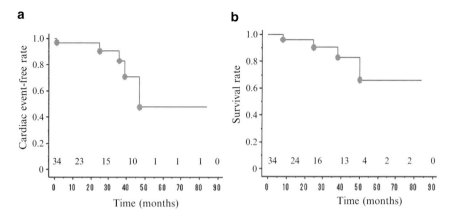

Fig. 1 (a) Cardiac event-free curve (Kaplan-Meier analysis), (b) Survival curve (Kaplan-Meier analysis)

Late cardiac events comprised 3 patients who underwent PCI for acute myocardial infarction arising from a new lesion, and 1 who was implanted with a pacemaker because of cardiac failure due to sick sinus syndrome. The mean follow-up duration was 25.2 ± 20.0 months. The three-year cardiac event free rate was 83.0% (Kaplan-Meier analysis) (Fig. 1a).

None of the patients died in hospital; the mean follow up duration was 28.6 ± 22.2 months and 4 non-cardiac late deaths occurred. The three-year survival rate was 90.6% (Kaplan-Meier analysis) (Fig. 1b).

Discussion

The incidence of patients with TAA combined with the coronary artery has increased with the increasing numbers of the elderly among the Japanese population and now ranges between 16 and 30% [1]. Simultaneous surgery reduces the postoperative risk of ischemic heart attack and the late cardiac mortality rate according to two studies [1,5].

Three patients in the present study who underwent postoperative PCI developed AMI from new lesions, but none had cardiac death. Thus, the outcomes of our simultaneous surgeries were satisfactory.

The prevention of postoperative cerebral infarction is essential to improve operative results. Our basic strategies for brain protection are the application of moderate to deep hypothermia during cross-clamping and maintaining brain perfusion with SCP. One patient had cerebral infarction and severe atherosclerotic plaque in the thoracic aorta. We carefully removed the atheromatous material around the ostium of the aortic arch branch and perfused the brain with SCP during the procedure. However, this patient developed a new cerebral infarction thereafter due to embolisms.

Some studies have indicated that simultaneous surgeries are associated with prolonged myocardial ischemia and CPB duration, which are considered significant risk factors for early mortality and morbidity [6,7]. We also emphasized the importance of careful strategic planning to minimize the duration of cardiopulmonary bypass and cardiac ischemia. The most important factor was performing CABG during core cooling and recovery from hypothermia. We completed as many of the planned graft–coronary artery anastomoses as possible during core cooling, and free grafts were used to infuse cardioplegic solution for myocardial protection.

Some authors prefer free grafts such as SVG and RA than *in situ* grafts for several reasons [3,8]. These include the fact that they can be used to infuse cardioplegic solution and because *in situ* graft flow such as LITA or RITA is dependent on subclavial artery flow and hemodynamic stability. Which of these grafts is optimal in these circumstances remains controversial. However, the excellent long-term patency of ITA and complete revascularization confer a survival benefit [9,10]. We used both free and *in situ* grafts to complete revascularization, performed LITA-LAD anastomosis during core cooling and restarted flow with re-beating of the heart. These strategies can minimize the duration of cardiac ischemia.

Conclusion

The early and late outcomes of simultaneous surgery for thoracic aortic aneurysm with coronary artery disease were satisfactory.

References

1. Kuniyoshi Y, Koja K, Miyagi K, et al (2002) Surgical treatment of aortic arch aneurysm combined with coronary artery stenosis. Ann Thorac Cardiovasc Surg 8:369–373
2. Narayan P, Rogers CA, Caputo M, et al (2007) Influence of concomitant coronary artery bypass graft on outcome of surgery of the ascending aorta/arch. Heart 93:232–237
3. Yamashiro S, Sakata R, Nakayama Y, et al (2001) One-stage thoracic aortic aneurysm treatment and coronary artery bypass grafting. Japan J Thoracic Cardiovasc Surg 49:236–243
4. Tamura N, Komiya T, Sakaguchi G, et al (2007) 'Turn-up' anastomotic technique for acute aortic dissection. Eur J Cardiothorac Surg 31:548–549
5. Tanaka T, Kazui T, Nakamura M, et al (1995) Surgical treatment of the true aortic arch aneurysm combined with coronary artery disease. Kyoubu Geka. 48:899–902
6. Ehrlich MP, Ergin MA, McCullough JN, et al (2000) Predictors of adverse outcome and transient neurologic dysfunction after ascending aorta/hemiarch replacement. Ann Thorac Surg 69:1755–1763
7. Sadahiro M, Niibori K, Tsuru Y, et al (1997) Risk factor analysis of early and late operative mortality after ascending aorta or aortic arch replacement. Ann Thorac Cardiovasc Surg 3:39–46

8. Kawashima T, Kazui T, Inoue N, et al (1993) Surgical treatment of the aortic arch aneurysm associated with coronary artery disease. Kyoubugeka 46:467–471
9. Ueda T, Shimizu H, Shin H, et al (2001) Detection and Management of concomitant coronary artery disease in patients undergoing thoracic aortic surgery. Jpn J Thorac Cardiovasc Surg 49:424–430
10. Cameron A, Davis KB, Green G, et al (1996) Coronary bypass surgery with internal-thoracic-artery grafts: effects on survival over a 15-year period. N Engl J Med 334:216–219

Svensson's (Modified Bentall) Technique using a Long Interposed Graft for Left Coronary Artery Reconstruction

Atsushi Nakahira, Yasuyuki Sasaki, Hidekazu Hirai,
Masanori Sakaguchi, Manabu Motoki, Shinsuke Kotani,
Koji Hattori, Toshihiko Shibata, and Shigefumi Suehiro

Backgrounds: Aortic root replacement remains challenging in coronary artery reconstructions.

Methods: From 1992, 40 patients (54.7±13.6 years; 4 with Marfan syndrome) underwent Svensson's technique, 11 of whom had histories of proximal aortic operations. The technique included coronary ostial reconstructions of the right with the buttons's technique and the left with a long interposed graft (8 or 10mm) anastomosed anteriorly in the composite graft. The technical advantages are unnecessary dissection around the left coronary artery, minimal tension and easy visualization of all anastomoses. Indications were annulo-aortic ectasia (n=26), acute/chronic aortic dissection (n=6 and 2), infective endocarditis (n=5) and aortic stenosis with porcelain aorta (n=1).

Results: After a mean 5.2 years, there were 2 hospital deaths of emergent cases and 6 late non-cardiac deaths. Patient's most recent echocardiograms showed the ejection fraction at 57.5±7.5 %. Coronary angiographies or enhanced computed tomographies performed in 26 patients (72%), at a mean of 3.1 years (range, 0.1–11.0) postoperatively, showed the patent interposed grafts. No complications associated with the interposed grafts or myocardial ischemia occurred.

Conclusions: The Svensson's technique was shown as justifiable with operative advantages, especially for complicated aortic roots, and good long-term patency of the interposed grafts without myocardial ischemic events.

A. Nakahira, Y. Sasaki, H. Hirai, M. Sakaguchi, M. Motoki, S. Kotani, K. Hattori, and S. Suehiro
Department of Cardiovascular Surgery, Osaka City University Graduate School of Medicine, Saitama, Japan

T. Shibata
Department of Cardiothoracic Surgery, Kansai Rosai Hospital, Saitama, Japan

Protective Effect on Preserved Aortic Valve Cusps of Reconstructed Pseudosinuses in the Aortic Root Reimplantation Technique

Kan Nawata, Shinichi Takamoto, Kansei Uno, Aya Ebihara, Tetsuro Morota, Minoru Ono, and Noboru Motomura

Summary

Background: Since 1998, we have experienced forty-three aortic root reimplantations. The former nineteen patients underwent so-called David I procedure (D1 group), and the latter twenty-four patients modified David V procedure (D5 group), in which pseudosinuses were reconstructed. Early outcomes of D5 group have been more satisfactory than that of D1 group.

Objective: To compare the root dimension and characteristic of the aortic valve motion after two types of reimplantation technique.

Methods: For twelve patients in D1 group and eighteen in D5 group, left ventricular dimension, aortic root diameter, and severity of aortic insufficiency were measured by transthoracic echocardiography (long axis view via left parasternal approach). Aortic valve motion was also investigated via M mode scan.

Results: Aortic annular diameter and left ventricular dimension were similar in both groups. Sinus of Valsalva was significantly larger in D5 group. Rapid valve opening/closing time, ejection time, maximal opening distance and opening distance just before rapid closing didn't show significant difference. Calculated rapid valve opening/closing velocity was the same, but slowly closing displacement before rapid valve closing was significantly larger in D5 group.

Conclusion: Slowly closing valve motion before rapid closing might contribute to the better valve durability in D5 group with pseudosinuses reconstruction.

K. Nawata, S. Takamoto, T. Morota, M. Ono, and N. Motomura
Department of Cardiothoracic Surgery

K. Uno and A. Ebihara
Department of Cardiovascular Medicine,
The University of Tokyo, Tokyo, Japan

K. Nawata (✉)
Hongo 7-3-1, Bunkyo-ku, Tokyo, 113-8655, Japan
e-mail: knawata-tky@umin.ac.jp

Keywords reimplantation · pseudosinus · valve leaflet motion · outcome · aortic root replacement

Background

Our primary strategy for patients with aortic root dilatation and normal aortic cusps is valve-sparing aortic root replacement. Since August, 1998 to October, 2007, we have experienced 44 cases of reimplantation technique. The first nineteen of them underwent David-I type reimplantation (original David-I: the D1 group), and the rest twenty-five patients underwent modified David-V type reimplantation (the D5 group). Early outcomes have been more satisfactory in the D5 group. Our modification of David-V reimplantation (UT modification) has been described before [1]. Shortly speaking, we use only one straight graft. To make pseudosinuses, one end of the graft is plicated at three triangular parts. Then the trimmed aortic root is reimplanted inside the tubular graft, securely tied onto the aortic root, sutured along the remnant cusps' line, and coronary buttons are anastomosed. Three longitudinal suture lines are made to make the tube narrow and the distal anasotomosis is done.

The profiles of the patients who underwent a reimplantation procedure are shown in Table 1. Operative outcomes after reimplantation are as shown in Tables 2a and 2b. Postoperative changes in aortic regurgitation after two types of reimplantation are demonstrated in Figure 1. The D1 group showed gradual progress or recur-

Table 1 Patients' profiles (Reimplantation)

	D1	D5	p value
n	19	25	–
Gender (Male:Female)	12:7	16:9	NS
Marfan Syndrome	15 (79%)	18 (72%)	NS
Age (years old)	31 ± 13	36 ± 16	NS
Valsalva sinus (mm)	55.5 ± 8.7	55.3 ± 8.4	NS
AR grade	1.6 ± 1.1	1.7 ± 1.4	NS
Follow-up (months)	58 ± 21	22 ± 14	<0.001

AR: aortic regurgitation

Table 2a Operative outcomes after reimplantation

mortality/morbidity	D1	D5
n	19	25
Hospital death	0	0
Remote death	4	1
(Suspected of rhythm death)	2	1
Major morbidity	3	3
(Major bleeding)	3	2
(Right heart failure)	0	1
AVR	4	1

AVR: aortic valve replacement

Table 2b NYHA (New York Heart Association Classification)

NYHA	D1	D5
I	15	24
II	3→AVR	0
III	0	0
IV	1→AVR	1→AVR

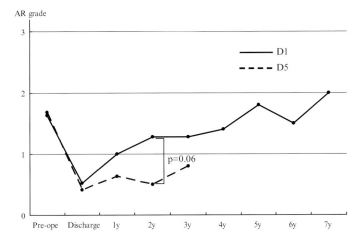

Fig. 1 Postoperative changes in aortic regurgitation after two different types of aortic reimplantation procedures

rence of aortic insufficiency after the operation. Though the number of the patients is small and the follow-up duration is short, the D5 group patients seemed to enjoy better outcome than the D1 group patients.

Objective

The purpose of this study is to compare the root dimension and characteristics of the aortic valve motion after two types of reimplantation technique, David-I (the D1 group) and modified David-V (the D5 group), and find out the protective factors on the valve durability after valve sparing aortic root replacement.

Patients and Methods

Postoperative follow-up examinations were available in 15 patients of D1 group and 19 patients of D5 group. Transthoracic echocardiography was performed by either of two specific cardiologists to evaluate left ventricular dimensions (long axis view), the grade of aortic regurgitation (AR), left ventricular outlet tract velocity (4 chamber view) and valve leaflet motions (M mode, Fig. 2) [2].

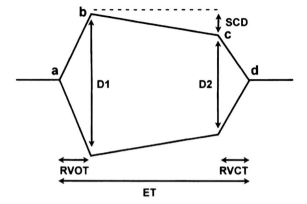

Fig. 2 Valve leaflet motions quoted from [2]
Values are obtained from M-mode of echocardiography. RVOT: Rapid Valve Opening Time, RVCT: Rapid Valve Closing Time, RVOV: Rapid Valve Opening Velocity, = D1/RVOT RVCV: Rapid Valve Closing Velocity, = D2/RVCT ET: Ejection time, D1: Maximum valve opening width, D2: Valve opening width just before rapid closing, SCD: Slowly Closing Displacement, = (D1-D2)/D1

Results

Data about aortic root dimensions, AR and valve leaflet motions are as shown in Tables 3a, 3b and 3c.

Discussions

In the D5 group, as we intended to make pseudosinuses, the estimated postoperative Valsalva sinus diameter was significantly larger than in the D1 group. This difference in aortic root dimensions didn't seem to affect global cardiac function or LV diameters. But, massive regurgitant flow through aortic valve seemed to influence the aortic valve leaflet motions and to lead to misinterpretation of the data, therefore, measured values from patients with grade 2 or 3 AR were excluded from the analysis of valve leaflet motions. Valve leaflet motions in the D5 group showed the equivalent maximal opening width and significantly larger slow closing displacement just before rapid valve closing, compared with the D1 group. This slow valve closing movement during the systolic phase seemed to contribute protectively to the better valve durability of the D5 group, and this valve motion is compatible to the larger vortex flow in significant pseudosinuses achieved in this group.

Table 3a Transthoracic echocardiography data (Aortic root dimension)

	D1	D5	p value
n	15	19	–
Preoperative AVD (mm)	25.6±2.4	25.4±2.5	NS
Postoperative AVD (mm)	20.2±1.3	20.3±1.9	NS
Postoperative Valsalva sinus (mm)	22.8±2.6	29.5±3.3	<0.0001
Postoperative Valsalva / AVD	1.13±0.08	1.47±0.22	0.0005
LVOT velocity (m/sec)	1.6±0.7	1.3±0.4	NS
LVDd (mm)	51.7±4.8	50.6±6.8	NS
LVDs (mm)	32.9±4.6	32.5±5.8	NS
LVEF	0.67±0.06	0.67±0.12	NS

AVD: aortic valve diameter
LVOT: left ventricular outlet tract
LVDd: left ventricular diameter in a diastolic phase
LVDs: left ventricular diameter in a systolic phase
LVEF: left ventricular ejection fraction

Table 3b Transthoracic echocardiography data (Aortic regurgitation)

AR grade	D1	D5
0	3	9
1	7	9
2	2	1
3	3	0
4	0	0

Patients with AR≧2 were excluded from the analysis of valve leaflet motions

Table 3c Transthoracic echocardiography data (Valve leaflet motions)

	D1	D5	p value
n	10	18	–
RVOT (msec)	35.3±16.3	33.8±10.8	NS
RVCT (msec)	45.5±16.0	44.9±18.3	NS
ET (msec)	339±49	324±70	NS
D1 (mm)	20.2±3.3	19.2±3.6	NS
D2 (mm)	18.8±3.1	16.1±3.8	0.03
SCD (%)	6.7±6.6	16.5±9.2	0.0015
RVOV (cm/sec)	70.6±44.1	61.8±16.2	NS
RVCV (cm/sec)	45.2±14.6	39.6±12.8	NS

Study Limitations

This study has some limitations. First, all of the operations examined here were performed by a single surgeon, and the operative outcomes might be affected by significant learning curve in the selection of patients and the surgeon's surgical technique. Secondly, the follow-up length is much different between the D1 and the D5 groups, and the influence of the secular change of valve leaflets on their motion might not be neglected, especially in the D1 group.

Conclusion

Creation of pseudosinuses in valve-sparing aortic root replacement contributed to the better valve leaflet motion, durability of the preserved valves and better clinical outcome.

References

1. Takamoto S, Nawata K, Morota T (2006) A simple modification of 'David-V' aortic root reimplantation. Eur J Cardiothorac Surg 30:560–562
2. Leyh RG, Schmidtke C, Sievers HH, et al (1999) Opening and closing characteristics of the aortic valve after different types of valve-preserving surgery. Circulation 100:2153–60

Modified Arch First Technique Using a Trifercated Graft

Seiichiro Wariishi, Hideaki Nishimori, Takashi Fukutomi, Kentaro Hirohashi, and Shiro Sasaguri

Objective: The arch first technique in the operation of total arch replacement for aortic arch aneurysms is advantageous to avoid neurological complication. We developed a *Modified Arch First Technique* using a hand-made trifurcated graft.

Methods: Thirteen patients were enrolled. A graft for reconstruction of arch vessels was prepared, which is consisted of a trunk (10 mm) and two branches (10 mm, 8 mm). Core cooling reached to 25°C. Arch vessels were serially reconstructed under unilateral cerebral perfusion through the right axillary artery before incising an aortic arch aneurysm. The antegrade cerebral perfusion was resumed through the trifurcated graft. Distal anastomosis was performed with another graft. A trifurcated graft was connected and proximal anastomosis was completed.

Results: There was 1 hospital death because of a residual thoraco-abdominal aortic aneurysm rupture. Morbidities were: reoperation for bleeding in 1 case and acute renal failure requiring hemodialysis in 2 cases, but no stroke occurred.

Conclusions: The modified arch first technique allows a simple and safe aortic arch replacement. A hand-made trifurcated graft is compact and offers a better operative field for distal anastomosis. It can minimize the risk of cerebral embolism by isolation of arch vessels from atheromas in aneurysm and reduction in cerebral ischemic time.

S. Wariishi, H. Nishimori, T. Fukutomi, K. Hirohashi, and S. Sasaguri
Department of Surgery II, Kochi University, Kochi, Japan

Atypical Arch Replacement

Reconstruction of Four Arch Vessels and Usefulness of Arch First Method with Combined Cerebral Perfusion

Takayuki Uchida, Hiromi Ando, Toru Yasutsune, Toshiro Iwai, Fumio Fukumura, and Jiro Tanaka

Abstract Recently, we experienced three atypical arch replacement cases. In these cases, we performed reconstruction of four arch vessels (because of anomaly of arch vessels). In such cases, it takes longer time for reconstruction of arch vessels. We used arch first technique with combined retro and partial-ante cerebral perfusion. Mean circulatory arrest time (including retrograde cerebral perfusion) was 44.3 ± 4.1(min),and Partial antegrade cerebral perfusion time was 21.5 ± 2.1 min. Postoperative courses were good. And there were no cerebral complication. Arch first technique with combined cerebral perfusion was thought to be safe and effective (for good operative field) method for atypical arch replacement.

Keywords anomaly of arch vessels · atypical arch replacement · arch first method · combined cerebral perfusion · cerebral protection

Introduction

We usually use arch first method (with deep hypothermia, circulatory arrest and retrograde cerebral perfusion (RCP)) for total arch replacement. Simple and bloodless operative field, and low incidence of cerebral embolism are the major advantages of this method. But the restriction of circulatory arrest time (or RCP time) is one of the major problems of this method.

Recently, we experienced three atypical arch replacement cases. We performed reconstruction of four arch vessels (because of anomaly of arch vessels) in these series. In such cases, it took longer time for reconstruction of arch vessels. So we used arch first technique with combined retro and partial-ante cerebral perfusion. (After reconstruction of lt.suclavian and lt.carotid artery with circulatory arrest or

T. Uchida (✉), H. Ando, T. Yasutsune, T. Iwai, F. Fukumura, and J. Tanaka
Department of Cardiovascular Surgery, Iizuka Hospital
e-mail: tuchidah1@aih-net.com

retrograde cerebral perfusion, residual arch vessel were clamped, and antegrade cerebral perfusion to left side arch vessels via graft was started. After completion of arch reconstruction, total antegrade cerebral perfusion via arch graft was started.)

Cases

We used our combined retro and partial-ante cerebral perfusion method for three atypical arch aneurysm cases.

In this method, canulation site was same as that of retrograde cerebral perfusion (femoral or ascending Aorta for arterial canulation, bicaval venous canulation). Under deep hypothermia (rectal temperature is below 20°C), we started arch reconstruction using branched graft and arch first technique. After finishing reconstruction of lt. suclavian and lt. carotid artery with circulatory arrest or retrograde cerebral perfusion, residual arch vessels were clamped, and antegrade cerebral perfusion to the left side arch vessels via graft was started. Then, pressure of rt. radial artery elevated to the half level of left side. After completion of arch reconstruction, total antegrade cerebral perfusion via arch graft was started. (Fig.1)

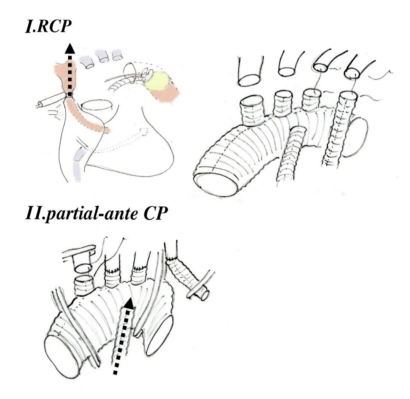

Fig. 1 Scheme of retro and partial-ante cerebral persuion. After reconstruction of lt.suclavian and lt.carotid artery, residual arch vessels are clamped, and partial-antegrade cerebral perfusion via graft is started

First case was 75 years old male, ruptured arch aneurysm combined with incomplete vascular ring (Fig. 2). The chief complaint was sudden onset back pain and dyspnea. Preoperative computed tomography revealed retroesophageal right subclavian artery. After aortotomy, we could see four orifices of arch vessels. We anastmosed 8 mm Hemashield to the fourth orifice (orifice of rt. SCA) first. Partial-antegrade cerebral perfusion via graft was started after reconstruction of lt. subclavian artery and lt. carotid artery. And after reconstruction of other three arch vessels, graft to fourth branch was anastmosed to the main branched graft. Fortunately, this patient had neither symptom of trachea compression nor cerebral complication after operation.

Second case was 79 years old female. The chief complaint was sudden onset chest and back pain. Diagnosis of this case was acute aortic dissection (Stanford A) combined with anomalous origin of lt. vertebral artery (originated directry form Aortic arch).

We found large entry at the aortic arch, and decided to perform total arch replacement. (Fig. 3)

This case was combined with Anomalous origin of lt vertebral artery. So we anastomosed 8 mm straight Hemashield graft to the lt.subclavian artery first. Stumps of lt. carotid artery and innnomanate artery was severely dissected. So we need stump plasity and took longer time before starting antegrade cerebral perfusion. (49 min) But postoperatively this patient had no cerebral damage, and discharged on foot.

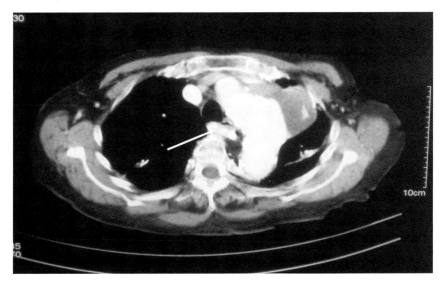

Fig. 2 Preoperative computed tomography of case1. Arrow indicates retroesophageal rt. subclavian artery originated directly form aortic arch

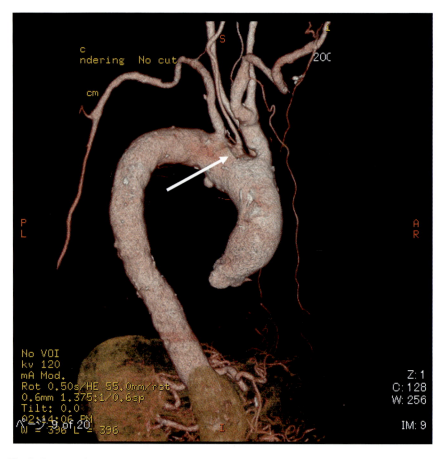

Fig. 3 Preoperative computed tomography of case3. Arrow indicates lt. vertebral artery originated directly from Aortic arch

The third case was 73 years old male with true arch aneurysm and anomalous origin of let vertebral artery. (This was only elective case.) So we performed the same operation with second case. We firstly anastomosed another 8 mm Hemashield to lt. subclavian artery. This graft was anastomosed to main branched graft finally. Post operative course was uneventful and this patient also discharged on foot.

Perioprative Results

During and partial-ante cerebral perfusion, average pressure of rt. radial artery (non perfusion site) during partial-antegrade cerebral perfusion was 35.5 (mmHg). And the average pressure of lt.radial artery (perfusion site) was 65.6 mmHg during this period.

RCP time was 44.3 ± 4.1(min), and Partial antegrade cerebral perfusion time was 21.5 ± 2.1 min. Postoperative courses were almost uneventful. Postoperative brain computed tomography showed no intracranial hypoperfuion in all cases. And all three cases had no neurological deficit and discharged on foot.

Discussion

We usually use arch first technique at total arch replacement, with retrograde cerebral perfusion (RCP). Bloodless simple and clear operative field is the first benefit of this method. And this method was reported improved both stroke and mortality rates in acute type A dissection cases by using arch first technique[1].

But the restriction of the RCP time is one of the major problem. Even though there is one case report of safety of RCP exceeding 120 min[2]. Ususially safty period of RCP is suggested to be about forty minutes.

Recently, Takamoto et al. reported the effectiveness of modified RCP method[3], but the techinique is relatively complicated. So we simply modificated the RCP method. (combined retro and partial-ante cerebral perfusion).

During partial ante CP, pressure of rt. Radial artery (non perfusion site) was about 50–60% of the other site. Clinically, this method was effective for extension of arch vessel reconstruction time.

Off course we know that we need more inspection and analysis about postoperative brain function about this method in more many cases from now on. And we also know our modificated method also has the limitation of perfuion duration. (Currently, we plan to perform selective cerebral perfusion from the beginning if we plan more than 90 min cerebral perfusion time preoperatively.)

But, in three cases, our modified RCP method was successful for atypical arch replacement. And we think this method is useful option of arch first technique.

References

1. Rokkas CK, Kouchoukos NT (1999) Single-stage extensive replacement of the thoracic aorta: the arch-first technique. J Thorac Cardiovasc Surg 117:99–104
2. Yamamoto S, Sasaguri, S, Fukuda T, et al (1998) Retrograde cerebral perfusion exceeding 120 minutes in aortic arch reconstruction: a report of two cases. Surg Today 28:98–101
3. Kitahori K, Takamoto S, Takayama H, et al (2005) A novel protocol of retrograde cerebral perfusion with intermittent pressure augmentation for brain protection. J Thorac Cardiovasc Surg 130:360–370

Distal Aortic Perfusion and Cerebrospinal Fluid Drainage for Thoracoabdominal Aortic Repair

Shinichi Suzuki, Kiyotaka Imoto, Keiji Uchida, Kensuke Kobayashi, Kouichiro Date, Motohiko Gouda, Toshiki Hatsune, Makoto Okiyama, Takayuki Kosuge, Yutaka Toyoda, and Munetaka Masuda

Summary

Objective: The purpose of this study was to evaluate the short-term results of thoracoabdominal repair using distal aortic perfusion and cerebrospinal fluid (CSF) drainage.

Methods: Between January 2000 and May 2007, we performed 38 thoracoabdominal aortic repairs. Twenty-five (66%) were male, and the mean age of all patients was 66 years, (range, 31 to 82 years). The patients distribution of thoracoabdominal aortic aneurysm, according to Safi's classification, was 8 extent I, 9 extent II, 7 extent III, 8 extent IV, and 6 extent V. Four patients, who presented with rupture underwent emergency repair. Distal aortic perfusion was used in 38 (100%) and CSF drainage in 14 (37%) of 38 patients.Twenty-nine (76%) of 38 patients inder-went intercostal artery reattachment.

Results: The hospital mortality was 16% (6 of 38 patinets), 9% (3 of 4 emergency repairs) and 9%(three of 34 non-emergency repairs). Immediate neurologic deficit was 2 (6%) of 38 patients, 1(25%) of 4 emergency repairs without CSF drainage, and 1(2.9%) of 34 non- emergency repairs.

Conclusions: The short-term results of thoracoabdominal repair using distal aortic perfusion, CSF drainage and aggressive intercostal aretery reattachment might be acceptable. But neurologic deficit following repairs of TAAA remains a devastating complication.

Keywords Thoracoabdominal aortic repair · Distal aortic perfusion · Cerebrospinal fluid drainage · Neurologic deficit · MD-CT

S. Suzuki, K. Imoto, K. Uchida, K. Kobayashi, K. Date, M. Gouda, T. Hatsune, M. Okiyama, T. Kosuge, Y. Toyoda, and M. Masuda
Yokohama City University School of Medicine, Cardiovascular Center

S. Suzuki (✉)
Yokohama City University School of Medicine, Cardiovascular Center
4-57 Urafune-cho, Minami-ku, Yokohama, Kanagawa 232-0024 Japan
e-mail: s-shin1@urahp.yokohama-cu.ac.jp

Introduction

The outcome of open repair of the thoracoabdominal aorta has steadily improved [1–11]. However neurological deficits (paraplegia and paraparesis) remain a serious complication associated with repair of the thoracoabdominal aorta.

Since 2000 we have used a combination of distal aortic perfusion and cerebrospinal fluid (CSF) drainage for repair of the thoracoabdominal aorta. The purpose of this study is to report the short-term results of repairs of the thoracoabdominal aorta.

Material and Methods

Patients

Between January 2000 and May 2007, we performed 38 thoracoabdominal aortic repairs. Twenty-five (66%) were male, and the mean age of all patients was 66 years, (range, 31 to 82 years). The distribution of thoracoabdominal aortic aneurysm(TAAA) in the patients, according to Safi's (modified Crawford's) classification (Fig.1) (2–4), was extent I, 8; extent II, 9; extent III, 7; extent IV, 8; and extent V, 6.

Primary indications were chronic dissection (20 patients, 52.6%), degenerative aneurysm (17 patients, 44.7%) and mycosis (1 patients, 2.6%).

Four patients, who presented with aortic rupture underwent emergency repair.

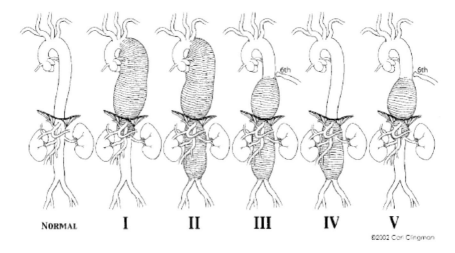

Fig. 1 Safi's (modified Crawford's) classification of thoracoabdominal aortic aneurysms

Surgical Technique

The patients were anesthetized and intubated, using a double-lumen endotracheal tube. Arterial catheters were placed in both upper and lower extremities and a pulmonary artery catheter was floated to allow continuous pressure monitoring. A transesophageal echo (TEE) probe was inserted into the esophagus. An epidural drain was placed percutaneously between the third and fourth lumbar space for monitoring cerebrospinal fluid (CSF) pressure and drainage in 14 of the 38 patients (37%). CSF pressure was maintained at less than 10 mmHg throughout the procedure. Motor evoked potentials (MEP) were used to monitor spinal cord function during surgery.

The patient was positioned in a right lateral decubitus position. The incision was tailored to complement the extent of the aneurysm (Fig. 1). The diaphragm was preserved, exposing the aortic hiatus and incising only the muscular portion of the diaphragm around the aorta. The patient was anticoagulated with heparin at a dose of 0.5 mg/Kg of body weight. The drainage tube was placed at right atrium through femoral vein or cannulated pulmonary artery for distal aortic perfusion. A centrifugal pump (Terumo Corp., Japan) with a heat exchanger and an oxygenator (Terumo Corp., Japan) was attached to the drainage tube and the arterial inflow was established through the common femoral artery.

Distal aortic perfusion was initiated just before applying the aortic clamp. For extensive aneurysms, sequential clamping was used. Patent lower intercostals arteries (T8-L2) were reattached, except in cases of heavily calcified or diseased aorta, or when technically not feasible. After completion of intercostal artery reattachment, the infrarenal abdominal aorta was clamped and the remainder of the aorta was opened. The visceral arteries were identified and perfused with blood via #10 or #12 SP stud catherters (Fuji systems Corp., Japan). Dacron grafts were used for repairs.

Postoperatively, CSF was drained intermittently by gravity to maintain a CSF pressure of less than 10 mmHg for 3 days.

Results

Surgical Mortality

The in-hospital mortality was 15.8% (6 of 38 patients) with 75% (3/4 patients) for emergency repair, and 8.8% (3/34 patients) for non-emergency repair.

The causes of the in-hospital mortality were necrosis of abdominal organs in 3 cases, respiratory failure in 1, and multiple organ failure due to infection in 2.

Neurologic Deficit

The incidence of neurologic deficit after all repairs was 5.2% (2 of 38 patients), with 25% (1 of 4 patients) for emergency repairs, and 2.9% (1 of 34 patients) for non-emergency repairs. CSF drainage could not be used for emergency repairs. Intercostal artery reattachment was performed in 76% of the patients (29 of 38 patients).

A Non-Emergent Case with Neurologic Deficit

The patient was 77 years old, extent III TAAA. Before the operation, aortogram the 11th intercostal artery was identified by aortogram, but the connection between the artery and anterior spinal artery was not found (Fig. 2).

The patient underwent open surgery for extent III TAAA. The 11th intercostal artery was not reattached because it was diseased around the ostia of the artery. After the surgery the patient suffered from paraplegia.

Recently, multidetecter computer tomography (MDCT) is used to evaluate the connection between intercostal arteries and anterior spinal artery (Fig. 3). If the connection between intercostal arteries and anterior spinal artery was identified in the patient, paraplegia might have been prevented.

Discussion

The open repair of the thoracoabdominal aorta is a challenging surgical procedure. Mortality form the surgery is still high and neurologic deficit following repair of TAAA remains a serious complication.

In Crawford's experience with 1,509 patients, aortic cross-clamp time greater than 60 minutes was associated with an incidence of paraplegia of 27% for the

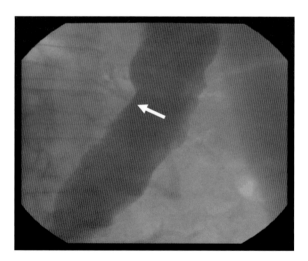

Fig. 2 Aortogram before the surgery; The 11th intercostal artery (white arrow)

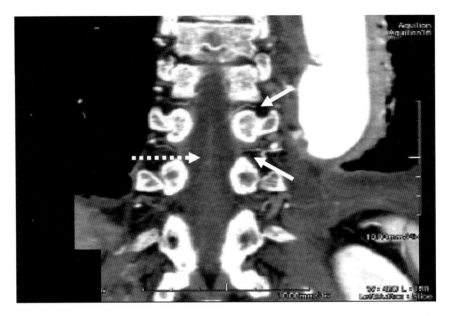

Fig. 3 Multidetecter computer tomography; Intercostal arteries (white arrows) and anterior spinal artery (white dotted arrow)

entire group, and when cases of extent II TAAA were specifically analyzed, the rate of paraplegia was as high as 50% [1].

Safi and colleagues hypothesized that by increasing distal aortic perfusion pressure using left heart bypass in combination with decreasing cerebrospinal fluid pressure with drainage, they could improve spinal cord perfusion and ultimately neurologic outcome during thoracoabdominal aortic repair. Since 1992 Safi and colleagues have used cerebrospinal fluid drainage, distal aortic perfusion, and passive moderate hypothermia with good success. In 1994, Safi and colleagues reported that neurologic deficit in patients treated for type I and type II TAAA was reduced significantly by perioperative cerebral spinal fluid drainage and distal aortic perfusion [2]. In 2001, Estrera and colleagues reported that with Safi's (modified Crawford's) classification of TAAA, extent III TAAA became significantly associated with neurologic deficit [6].

Since 2000, we introduced CSF drainage for repair of TAAA. From the beginning it has been used in patients at high risk with extent I and II TAAA. And since 2003 we have used CSF drainage in patients with extent III TAAA. In our series, the incidence of neurologic deficit after all repairs was 5.2% (2 of 38 patients), which might be thought acceptable. Two patients who suffered from neurologic deficit had extent III TAAA. CSF drainage could not been used in one of them, because the cause of the TAAA was active infection and the patient was hemodynamically unstable. We have not used CSF drainage in patients with extent IV and V TAAA, because the incidence of neurologic deficit with extent IV and V TAAA might be low. There was no neurologic deficit in patients with extent IV and V TAAA in our series.

In the last decade major advances in the use of adjuncts (distal aortic perfusion and CSF drainage), surgical techniques, and anesthesia have reduced mortality and complications in patients undergoing thracoabdominal and descending thoracic aortic aneurysm surgery [5–11]. In 2005, Safi and colleagues reported that the overall incidence of neurologic deficit was 3.3% (36 of 1,106). Though the adjunct use during repair of the thoracoabdominal aorta significantly reduced the risk of neurologic deficit, despite increasing aortic cross-clamp time, neurological deficit (paraplegia and paraparesis) remains a serious complication associated with repairs of thoracoabdominal aorta.

To avoid neurological deficit, preoperative visualization of the spinal cord blood supply has been suggested and used [12–16]. Magnetic resonance angiography (MRA) [12,14,15] and computed tomography angiography (CTA) [13,15,16] have been explored to investigate their potential to localize the Adamkiewicz artery and its segmental supplier. Detection rate of the Adamkiewicz artery varies from 69% to 97% for MRA [12,14,15] and from 71% to 92 % for CTA [13,15,16]. In 2007, Saito reported [16] at the AATS annual meeting that selective reconstruction of the preoperatively identified Adamkiewicz artery during repair of descending or thoracoabdominal aortic aneurysm is effective for maintaining blood flow to the spinal cord to prevent neurologic deficit.

In 2005, we started to use CTA to identify the Adamkiewicz artery before and after surgery. We believe that preoperative detection of the Adamkiewicz artery will result in a decrease in postoperative neurological deficit.

The limitation of this study was that it was a retrospective analysis and number of patients was small. A large-scale prospective randomized clinical controlled study is necessary.

Conclusion

In conclusion, the short-term results of thoracoabdominal repair using distal aortic perfusion, CSF drainage, and aggressive intercostal aretery reattachment are acceptable, but neurologic deficit following repair of TAAA remains a serious complication.

References

1. Svensson LG, Crawford ES, Hess KR, et al (1993) Experience with 1509 patients undergoing thoracoabdominal aortic operations. J Vasc Surg 17:357–68 (discussion368–70)
2. Safi HJ, Bartoli S, Hess KR, et al (1994) Neurologic deficit in patients at high risk with thoracoabdominal aortic aneurysms: the role of cerebral spinal fluid drainage and distal aortic perfusion. J Vasc Surg 20:434–44 (discussion 442–3)

3. Safi HJ, Hess KR, Randel M, et al (1996) Cerebrospinal fluid drainage and distal aortic perfusion: reducing neurologic complications in repair of thoracoabdominal aortic aneurysm type I and II. J Vasc Surg 23: 223–8 (discussion 229)
4. Safi HJ, Campbell MP, Miller CC 3rd, et al (1997) Cerebral spinal fluid drainage and distal aortic perfusion decrease the incidence of neurological deficit: the results of 343 descending and thoracoabdominal aortic aneurysm repairs. Eur J Vasc Edovasc Surg 14:118–24
5. Safi HJ, Campbell MP, Ferreira ML, et al (1998) Spinal cord protection in descending thoracic and thoracoabdominal aortic aneurysm repair. Semin Thorac Cardiovasc Surg 10:41–4
6. Estrera AL, Miller CC 3rd, Huynh TT, et al (2001) Neurologic outcome after thoracic and thoracoabdominal aortic aneurysm repair.(2001) Ann Thorac Surg 72:1225–30.(discussion 1230–1)
7. Estrera AL, Rubenstein FS, Miller CC 3rd, et al (2001) Descending thoracic aortic aneurysm: surgical approach and treatment using the adjuncts cerebrospinal fluid drainage and distal aortic perfusion. Ann Thorac Surg 72:481–6
8. Huynh TT, Miller CC 3rd, Estrera AL, et al (2002) Determinants of hospital length of stay after thoracoabdominal aortic aneurysm repair. J Vasc Surg 35: 648–53
9. Safi HJ, Miller CC 3rd, Huynh TT, et al (2003) Distal aortic perfusion and cerebrospinal fluid drainage for thoracoabdominal and descending thoracic aortic repair. Ten years of organ protection. Ann Surg 238:372–381
10. Suzuki S, Davis III CA, Miller CC 3rd, et al (2003) Cardiac function predicts mortality following thoracoabdominal and descending thoracic aortic aneurysm repair. Eur J Cardiothorac Surg 24:119–124
11. Safi HJ, Estrera AL, Miller CC 3rd, et al (2005) Evolution of risk for neurologic deficit after descending and thoracoabdominal aortic repair. Ann Thorac Surg 80:2173–9
12. Yamada N, Okita Y, Minatoya K, et al (2000) Preoperative demonstration of the Adamkiewicz artery by magnetic resonance angiography in patients with descending or thoracoabdominal aortic aneurysms. Eur J Cardiothorac Surg 18:104–11
13. Takase K, Sawamura Y, Igarashi K, et al (2002) Demonstration of the artery of Adamkiewicz at multi-detector row helical CT. Radiology 223:39–45
14. Hyodoh H, Kawaharada N, Akiba H, et al (2005) Usefulness of preoperative detection of artery of Adamkiewicz with dynamic contrast-enhanced MR angiography. Radiology 236:1004–1009
15. Nijenhuis RJ, Jacobs MJ, Jaspers K, et al (2007) Comparison of magnetic resonance with computed tomography angiography for preoperative localization of the Adamkiewicz artery in thoracoabdominal aortic aneurysm patients. J Vasc Surg 45:677–85
16. Saito S, Aomi S, Tomioka H, et al (2007) Development of collateral blood supply for spinal cord immediately after descending or thoracoabdominal repair with selective reconstruction of Adamkiewicz artery. Presented at the 87th annual meeting of American association for Thoracic Surgery

Selective Reconstruction of Preoperatively Identified Adamkiewicz Artery During Descending and Thoracoabdominal Aortic Aneurysm Repair; What we have Learned

Satoshi Saito, Shigeyuki Aomi, Hideyuki Tomioka, Masayuki Miyagishima, and Hiromi Kurosawa

Paraparesis and paraplegia after repair of the descending (TAA) or thoracoabdominal (TAAA) repair remains devastating complication. The purpose of this study was to determine the effects of selective reconstruction of Adamkiewicz artery (ARM) preoperatively identified with MDCT upon neurological outcome.

Methods: Sixty two consecutive patients who had aneurysms of the descending (n=15) or thoracoabdominal aorta (n=47) were studied prospectively with MDCT to identify ARM before and after surgery. Median age was 62 years (29 to 77) and 37 patients had non-dissecting aneurysm and 23 had aortic dissections. The repair was performed and the segmental intercostals arteries (ICA) connected with ARM were reconstructed selectively according to the identification of ARM with MDCT.

Results: MDCT demonstrated the ARM in 57 (91.9%) of the 62 patients. The hospital deaths occurred in 3 patients (4.8%). No paraplegia but 1 paraparesis (1.6 %) occurred in a patients. Major different source of blood supply was identified in 18 (34.6%), and 12/58 (20.6%) reconstructed arteries were occluded with other collateral development.

Conclusion: Selective reconstruction of ARM during repair of thoracoabdominal aortic aneurysm is safe and effective reducing the incidence of neurological deficit. Collateral blood supply for spinal cord develops postoperatively and the considerations of collateral source is crucially important.

S. Saito, S. Aomi, H. Tomioka, M. Miyagishima, and H. Kurosawa
Tokyo Women's Medical University, Tokyo, Japan

Poster Session 3
Miscellaneous

Three-stage Monitoring for Prevention of Cerebral Malperfusion During Cardiovascular Surgery

Kazumasa Orihashi, Taijiro Sueda, Kenji Okada, and Katsuhiko Imai

Summary We present our current strategy for preventing cerebral malperfusion during cardiovascular surgery, "three-stage monitoring", that consists of: 1) near-infrared spectroscopy for continuously monitoring regional oxygen saturation in frontal lobes; 2) orbital Doppler to measure central retinal arterial flow (representing carotid artery perfusion); and 3) transesophageal echocardiography for elucidating the cause of malperfusion. Consecutive 358 cases were divided into two groups: 203 cases after establishment of monitoring and 155 cases before establishment. Cerebral infarction and transient events were examined in both groups. There were 10 cases of infarction (2.8%) and 45 cases of transient events (12.6%). After monitoring was established, events decreased from 21.9% to 10.3% (p=0.0026). Incidence of infarction decreased from 3.9% to 2.0% and transient events decreased from 18.1% to 8.4% (p=0.0061). Drop in regional oxygen saturation alerted an occurrence of malperfusion, orbital Doppler confirmed it, and transesophageal echocardiography revealed its mechanism and suggested solutions. What is important to prevent neurological sequelae, not only detection of malperfusion but information on the cause is important because measures needs to be taken toward early recovery of cerebral perfusion before damage becomes irreversible. Three stage monitoring may benefit for this purpose.

Keywords aortic dissection · cerebral malperfusion · transesophageal echocardiography · near-infrared spectroscopy

---

K. Orihashi, T. Sueda, K. Okada, and K. Imai
Division of Cardiovascular Surgery, Hiroshima University Hospital

K. Orihashi (✉)
Division of Cardiovascular Surgery, Hiroshima University Hospital
Kasumi 1-2-3, Minami-ku, Hiroshima, 734-8551 Japan
e-mail: orichan@hiroshima-u.ac.jp

Introduction

Two mechanisms are responsible for neurological damage during cardiovascular surgery: embolism and sustained malperfusion. While the former is related to the surgical procedure or extracorporeal circulation and is irreversible, the latter can be avoided by early detection and appropriate restoration of cerebral perfusion. Three-stage monitoring was established for dealing with cerebral malperfusion. It consists of: 1) near-infrared spectroscopy (NIRS) for continuously monitoring regional oxygen saturation in the frontal lobes; 2) orbital Doppler to measure central retinal arterial flow (representing carotid arterial perfusion); and 3) transesophageal echocardiography (TEE) for elucidating the cause of malperfusion. In this report, we describe the methods used for three-stage monitoring and the short-term outcome when this type of monitoring is used in patients undergoing cardiovascular surgery.

Materials and Methods

For NIRS monitoring, TOS-96 (TOSTEC Co. Ltd, Tokyo, Japan) was used [1]. Oxygen saturation was continuously monitored in the bilateral anterior lobe (rSO2) throughout surgery. When the rSO2 dropped within minutes, reduced cerebral blood flow was considered the most likely mechanism if there was no decrease in oxygenation of arterial blood. In such instances, orbital Doppler was employed to assess cerebral perfusion.

For orbital Doppler, a conventional 7.5 MHz sector transducer (used conventionally for precordial echocardiography) was placed on the eyelid and horizontally scanned [2]. The color signal of the central retinal artery was detected in the echo image beneath the optic disk. The flow velocity was normally several cm/sec during systole. When the color signal became undetectable with orbital Doppler, malperfusion was strongly suspected. TEE was then employed to identify the reason for malperfusion.

The arch branches were visualized on TEE as reported previously [3]. Based on the information provided by TEE, a course of action was determined to correct the cerebral malperfusion. The adequacy of the corrective action was then examined with NIRS and orbital Doppler.

Three-hundred-fifty-eight consecutive cases undergoing cardiovascular surgery were examined. The surgical procedures were CABG, valvular surgery, aortic surgery, and others in 131, 114, 87, and 26 cases, respectively. These cases were divided into two groups: 155 and 203 cases before and after establishment of 3-stage monitoring. The incidence of neurological events was compared regarding: 1) cerebral infarction, and 2) transient events such as delirium, anisocoria, involuntary movements, which were determined from the chart.

Results

The results are listed in Table 1. The total incidence of neurological events significantly decreased after establishment of 3-stage monitoring. In the breakdown of total events, transient events significantly decreased, while there was a decrease in cerebral infarction that did not reach statistical significance.

Three illustrative cases are presented. In two cases, malposition of the selective cerebral perfusion catheter led to cerebral malperfusion. NIRS was useful for detecting the onset of malperfusion, which was confirmed by orbital Doppler. In addition, TEE identified the reason for malperfusion in these cases. When the catheter position was corrected, cerebral perfusion was restored as shown by NIRS and orbital Doppler.

Another case had aortic dissection that extended into all three arch branches. A true lumen in the innominate artery was narrowed by an expanded false lumen. Right axillary perfusion was started in expectation that the increased perfusion pressure would restore the true lumen in the innominate artery. However, it led to hypoperfusion of the left hemisphere and the body. Left axillary perfusion was added and improved perfusion was immediately confirmed by NIRS and orbital Doppler.

Discussion

In order to prevent neurological complications, it is important to detect the onset of malperfusion and to identify its cause, because cerebral perfusion needs to be restored before neuronal damage becomes irreversible.

From our results, three-stage monitoring appears to be feasible and effective. NIRS continuously and noninvasively provides real-time information on oxygen debt in the brain and is suitable for detecting the onset of unexpected malperfusion. Orbital Doppler assesses flow in the central retinal artery and is useful for the confirmation of flow reduction in the carotid artery. As shown in the illustrative cases, TEE is capable of visualizing events in the arch vessels in real time and

Table 1 Results of three-stage monitoring

Period n	Before 155	After 203	Total 358	
Events	34	21	55	
	(21.9%)	(10.3%)	(14.2%)	p = 0.0026
Infarction	6	4	10	
	(3.9%)	(2.0%)	(2.8%)	p = 0.4487
Transient	28	17	45	
	(18.1%)	(8.4%)	(12.6%)	p = 0.0061

provides morphological and hemodynamic information. Although some technical expertise is needed for visualization, TEE is beneficial for making decisions that can rapidly restore cerebral perfusion. Our results show that unexpected events may occur that are not always visible in the operative field.

References

1. Orihashi K, Sueda T, Okada K, et al (2004) Near-infrared spectroscopy for monitoring cerebral ischemia during selective cerebral perfusion. Eur J Cardio-thorac Surg 26:907–911
2. Orihashi K, Matsuura Y, Sueda T, et al (2001) Clinical implication of orbital ultrasound monitoring during selective cerebral perfusion. Ann Thorac Surg 71:673–7
3. Orihashi K, Matsuura Y, Sueda T, et al (2000) Aortic arch branches are no longer blind zone for transesophageal echocardiography: a new eye for aortic surgeons. J Thorac Cardiovasc Surg 120:466–72

Induction of Phosphorylated BAD in Motor Neurons After Transient Spinal Cord Ischemia in Rabbits

Masahiro Sakurai, Koji Abe, Yasuto Itoyama, and Koichi Tabayashi

Summary The mechanism of spinal cord injury has been thought to be related to the vulnerability of spinal motor neuron cells against ischemia. We previously reported that spinal motor neurons might be lost by programmed cell death, and investigated a possible mechanism of neuronal death by immunohistochemical analysis for Phosphorylated Bad (P-Bad) and Bad. We employed rabbit spinal cord ischemia model with an use of balloon catheter. The spinal cord was removed at 8 hours, 1, 2, or 7 days after 15 min of transient ischemia, and western blot analysis for P-Bad and Bad and double-label fluorescence immunocytochemical studies were performed. Western blot analysis revealed no immunoreactivity for P-Bad and Bad in the sham-operated spinal cords. However, they became apparent at 8 hours after transient ischemia, which returned to the baseline level at 1 day. Double-label fluorescence immunocytochemical study revealed that both P-Bad and Bad were positive at 8 hours of reperfusion in the same motor neurons which eventually die. These results suggest that transient spinal cord ischemia activates both cell death and survival pathways after ischemia. The induction of P-Bad protein at the early stage of reperfusion may be one of the factor responsible for the delay in neuronal death after spinal cord ischemia.

Keywords spinal cord ischemia · Phosphorylated Bad · motor neuron death

---

K. Abe
Department of Cardiovascular Surgery
National Hospital Organization Sendai Medical Center, Sendai Japan

Y. Itoyama
Department of Neurology,
Okayama University Graduate School of Medicine, Okayama, Japan

K. Tabayashi
Departments of Neurology and [4]Cardiovascular Surgery
Tohoku University Graduate School of Medicine, Sendai, Japan

M. Sakurai, (✉)
Department of Cardiovascular Surgery, National Hospital Organization Sendai Medical Center
2-8-8, Miyagino, Miyagino-ku, Sendai, 983-8520 Japan
e-mail: sakuraim@snh.go.jp

Spinal cord injury after a successful operation of thoracic aorta is a disastrous complication in humans. However, the exact mechanism of such delayed vulnerability is not fully understood. In rabbit spinal cord ischemia model, we have reported delayed and selective motor neuron death after transient ischemia [1,2]. Furthermore in this model, we have reported that delayed and selective motor neuron death was greatly associated with an activated apoptotic signals of the caspase3 cascade and we have also reported that immunoreactivities for both Akt and caspase3 were induced at the early stage of reperfusion in the same motor neuron which eventually die [2]. To evaluate the mechanism of such selective vulnerability of motor neurons, we attempted to make a reproducible model for spinal cord ischemia, and analyzed cell damage.

Bad is one of the downstream factors of the Akt pathway, and a proapoptotic member of the Bcl-2 family that can displace Bax from binding to Bcl-2 and Bcl-xL, resulting in cell death [3,4] Survival factors such as IL-3 can inhibit the apoptotic activity of Bad by activating intracellular signaling pathways that result in the phosphorylation of Bad at serine-112 and serin-136 [4]. Phosphorylation at these sites results in the binding of Bad to 14-3-3 proteins and the inhibition of Bad binding to Bcl-2 and Bcl-xL [4]. Akt has been shown to promote cell survival by its ability to phosphorylate Bad at serine-136 [5,6]. Although it has not been shown Bad works after spinal cord ischemia, Bad and P-Bad signaling pathway may be important for neuronal survival. To understand cell death mechanisms after spinal cord ischemia, we investigated the cell death and survival pathways in motor neurons after transient spinal cord ischemia.

During the experiment, the animals were treated in accordance with the declaration of Helsinki and the guiding principles in the care and use of animals. Also, the experimental and animal care protocol was approved by the animal care committee of Tohoku University School of Medicine.

Twenty-five domesticated white rabbits, in Japan, weighing 2 to 3 kg were used in this study and divided into two groups: a 15 minutes ischemia, and a sham control groups. We employed rabbit spinal cord ischemia model with an use of balloon catheter according to our previous method. Animals were allowed to recover at an ambient temperature, and were sacrificed at 8 h and 1, 2, and 7 days after the reperfusion (n=5 at each time point). The tissue samples for histological and immunohistochemical studies were frozen in powdered dry ice and stored at −80°C.

In order to investigate changes of P-Bad and Bad expression, we performed Western blot analysis according to our previous method with use the primary antibodies: sheep polyclonal anti-P-Bad (ser136) antibody (B5804; Sigma, Saint Louis, Missouri, USA) and goat polyclonal anti-Bad (N19) antibody (SC-6542; Santa Cruz Biotechnology, Inc., California, CA, USA).

We also performed fluorescence double-labeling study to investigate colocalization of P-Bad and Bad according to our previous method with use the primary antibodies : donkey anti-goat lgG linked with TexasRed I : 50 (705-075-147, Jackson Immunoreseach, PA, U.S.A.) and donkey anti-sheep lgG linked with fluo-rescein (FITC) I : 50 (713-095-147, Jackson Immunoreseach, PA, U.S.A.). The slides were mounted in aqueous mounting media with DABCO and observed using fluorescein microscopy. Quantitative analyses of the neurological score, the cell numbers, and the optical density of Western blots were analyzed by ANOVA. p value less than 0.05 was considered statistically significant. Parametric data are present as mean ± S.D.

Representative results of Western blot analysis are shown in Fig. 1. With antibody against P-Bad, no band was detectable in samples of sham control, but those at 8 hours after blood flow restoration revealed a single band with molecular weight of 23 kDa (Fig. 1, upper, left). With antibody against Bad, no band was detectable in samples of sham control, but those at 8 hours after blood flow restoration revealed a single band with molecular weight of 25 kDa (Fig. 1, upper right). This band became scarcely detectable at 1 day after reperfusion. This band became scarcely detectable at 1 day after reperfusion. The membrane without the primary antibody revealed no band (data not shown). With quantitative analysis, we found that P-Bad and Bad were significantly increased at 8 hours of reperfusion (*$p < 0.0001$, **$p < 0.0001$) (Fig. 1, lower).

The results of P-Bad and Bad double-staining immunohistochemistry are shown in Fig.2. P-Bad was strongly colocalized with Bad in motor neurons at only 8 hours of reperfusion. Furthermore,, about 85% of motor neurons expressed both P-Bad and Bad (Fig. 2).

We have previously demonstrated delayed and selective motor neuron death in lumbar regions of the rabbit spinal cord with the same reproducible model [1,2].

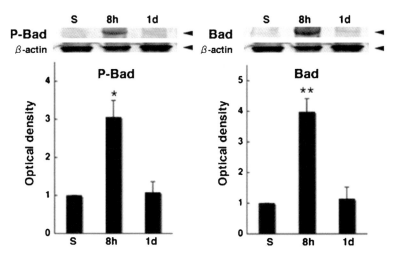

Fig. 1 Representative Western blot for P-Bad and Bad. Immunoreactivity was only weakly (P-Bad) or was not (Bad) detected in sham-controls (S). Strong bands are observed at the expected size (23 kD and 25 kD, respectively) at 8 hours (8 h) after blood flow restoration, but became less dense at 1 day (1 d). β-actin showed no change. Quantitative analysis showed that 15 minutes ischemia significantly increased P-Bad and Bad at 8 hours of reperfusion (*$p < 0.0001$, **$p < 0.0001$ compared with sham control group and reperfusion at 1 day group)

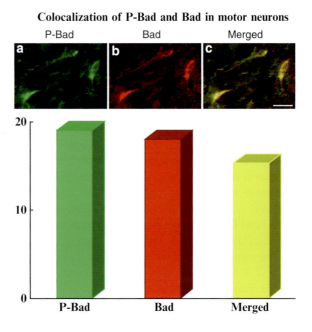

Fig. 2 Co-localization of P-Bad and Bad in motor neurons at 8 hours after ischemia. P-Bad was detected by fluorescein isothiocyanat (green) (A), and Bad by Texas red (red) (B). The merged image is shown in (C) with double positive as yellow color. Bar=50μm. Quantitative analysis showed that about 85% of motor neurons expressed both P-Bad and Bad

Fifteen minutes of ischemia is a relatively short period in comparison to those of previously reported ischemic models [7]. After the ischemia, delayed and selective motor neuron damage was observed only after 7 days of reperfusion, a phenomenon known as selective neuronal death in motor neuron cells after spinal cord ischemia [1,2,8] similar to the delayed selective neuronal death in hippocampal CA1 cells after cerebral ischemia. This result shows that motor neuron cells are most vulnerable to spinal ischemic injury.

Recently, report has described that decreases in P-Bad and Bad/14-3-3 dimerization and increases in Bcl-xL/Bad and Bcl-2/Bad dimerization observed after rat brain ischemia, were prevented by SP600125 administration. These results suggest that Bad may be an integrated checkpoint of the survival and death signaling and that it contributes to cell fate after rat brain ischemia. [9] In this study, the increase in the immunoreactivity of both P-Bad and Bad were demonstrated selectively in ventral motor neuron cells in the spinal cord after 8 hours of reperfusion. Therefore, the mechanism of cell injury of the motor neurons in the spinal cord and the cells of the brain after ischemia may similar.

A recent study showed that level of Bad in the spinal cord of early symptomatic and end stage transgenic mutant SOD mice were dramatically higher than those in controls. In nontransgenic and asymptomatic transgenic mSOD1 mice, most, if not all, available Bax and Bad are neutralized through phosphorylation and binding to Bcl-2 and Bcl-xL, resulting in a molecular equilibrium that favors cell survival. Conversely, during the neurodegenerative process there is an increased formation of Bax and un phosphorylated Bad, resulting in a new molecular equilibrium that favor cell death in this model of ALS. [10] In this study, the increase in the immunoreactivity of Bad was demonstrated selectively in ventral motor neuron cells in the spinal cord after 8 hours of reperfusion. This finding suggests that the oxidative injury could activate cytokines and augment Bad activity as compensatory mechanism. Therefore, our results suggest that the mechanism of motor neuron death in the spinal cord after ischemia might have a similar feature with that of ALS.

This study also demonstrates that immunoreactivities for both Bad and P-Bad were induced at 8 hours in the same motor neuron, which eventually die. These results suggest that transient spinal cord ischemia activates both cell death and survival pathways after ischemia. The activation of P-Bad protein at the early stage of reperfusion may be one of the factor responsible for the delay in neuronal death after spinal cord ischemia.

References

1. Sakurai M, Nagata T, Abe K, et al (2003) Survival- and death promoting events after transient spinal cord ischemia in rabbits: induction of Akt and caspase3 in motor neurons. J Thorac Cardiovasc Surg 125:370–377
2. Sakurai M, Takahashi G, Abe K, et al (2005) Endoplasmic reticulum stress induced in motor neurons by transient spinal cord ischemia in rabbits. J Thorac Cardiovasc Surg 130: 640–645
3. Yang E, Zha J, Jokel J, et al (1995) Bad, a heterodimeric partner for Bcl-XL and Bcl-2, displaces Bax and promotes cell death. Cell 80: 285–291
4. Zha J, Harada H, Yang E, et al (1996) Serine phosphorylation of death agonist BAD in response to survival factor results in binding to 14-3-3 not BCL-X(L). Cell 87: 619–628
5. Datta SR, Dudek H, Tao X, et al (1997) Akt phosphorylation of BAD couples survival signal to the cell-intrinsic death machinery. Cell 91:231–241
6. del Peso L, Gonzalez-Garcia M, Page C, et al (1997) Interleukin-3-induced phosphorylation of BAD through the protein kinase Akt. Science 278: 687–689
7. Herold JA, Kron IL, Langenburg SE, et al (1994) Complete prevention of postischemic spinal cord injury by means of regional infusion with hypothermic saline and adenosine. J Thorac Cardiovasc Surg 107:536–42
8. DeGirolami U, Zivin JA (1982) Neuropathology of experimental spinal cord ischemia in the rabbit. J Neuropathol Exp Neurol 41: 129–149
9. Kamada H, Nito C, Endo H, et al (2007) Bad as a converging signaling molecule between survival PI3 = K/Akt and death JNK in neurons after transient focal cerebral ischemia in rats. J Cereb Blood Floe Metab 27:521–533
10. Vukosavic S, Dubois-Dauphin M, Romero N, et al (1999) Bax and Bcl-2 interaction in a transgenic mouse model of familial amyotrophic lateral sclerosis. J. Neurochem. 73:2460–2468

Modifying Anastomotic Site in Thoracic Aortic Surgery by Using Biodegradable Felt Strips With or Without Basic Fibroblast Growth Factor

Hidenori Fujiwara, Yoshikatsu Saiki, Katsuhiko Oda, Satoshi Kawatsu, Ichiro Yoshioka, Naoya Sakamoto, Toshiro Ohashi, Masaaki Sato, Yasuhiko Tabata, and Koichi Tabayashi

Objectives: The purposes of this investigation are to elucidate sequelae of reinforcing the anastomotic site with nonbiodegradable PTFE felt, biodegradable polyglycol acid (PGA), and PGA with basic fibroblast growth factor (bFGF) in a thoracic aortic replacement model.

Methods: Replacement of the descending thoracic aorta was performed in beagles (n = 19) using the above three different materials or without reinforcement (control).

Results: The medial thickness in the PTFE group was significantly lower than that of the PGA with bFGF group (66±5% versus 90±4% of control, < 0.05). The adventitial layer in the PTFE group significantly decreased in thickness compared to control (42±8% of control, <0.05), whereas those in the PGA and PGA with bFGF groups significantly thickened (117±11 and 134±14% of control, respectively, < 0.05), which was associated with increased vessel number. The failure force measured at anastomotic sites did not show statistical difference between the four groups.

Conclusions: The aortic wall at the anastomotic site reinforced with nonbiodegradable felt showed thinning of both media and adventitia. These changes were associated with diminished vessels in the adventitial layer. Biodegradable felt with or without bFGF reversed these histological changes without altering biomechanical strength.

H. Fujiwara, Y. Saiki, K. Oda, S. Kawatsu, I. Yoshioka, and K. Tabayashi
Department of Cardiovascular Surgery, Tohoku University Graduate School of Medicine, Sendai, Japan

N. Sakamoto, T. Ohashi, and M. Sato
Tohoku University Graduate School of Mechanical Engineering, Japan

Y. Tabata
Institute for Frontier Medical Science, Kyoto, Japan

Late Outcome of Extra-anatomic Bypass for Infected Abdominal Aortic Aneurysm

Atsushi Tabuchi, Hisao Masaki, Yasuhiro Yunoki, Takuro Yukawa, Hiroshi Kubo, Eiichiro Inagaki, Sohei Hamanaka, and Kazuo Tanemoto

We examined the surgical result and late outcome of the extra-anatomic bypass for infected abdominal aortic aneurysm. Seven patients underwent operations in our institution and were male with a mean age of 68.4 years. Our surgical procedure was an extra-anatomic bypass grafting (axillo-bilateral femoral bypass). There was a resection of the aneurismal wall and debridement of all infected tissue. Aortic and iliac arterial stumps were closed by direct sutures and covered by the greater ometum. The post-operative early complications were an aortic stump disruption due to retroperitoneal abscess in one patient. There were no hospital deaths. The late outcome was a left renal abscess in one patient and he underwent a left nephrectomy and drainage 14 months after his operation. The unilateral bypass graft occlusion occurred in the bilateral axillo-femoral bypass grafting, and he underwent femoro-femoral crossover bypass grafting 12 months after his operation. Late death occurred with one patient due to cerebral vascular disease and other patients continued follow-up examinations 15 to 132 months after their operations. No one had aortic stump disruption, recurrence of infected aneurysm and/or limb ischemia. We concluded that the extra-anatomic bypass for infected abdominal aortic aneurysm was a safe and excellent method.

A. Tabuchi, H. Masaki, Y. Yunoki, T. Yukawa, H. Kubo, E. Inagaki, S. Hamanaka, and K. Tanemoto
Division of Thoracic and Cardiovascular Surgery, Department of Surgery, Kawasaki Medical School, Kurashiki, Japan

The Efficacy of a Bionic Baroreflex System in an Abdominal Aortic Aneurysm Surgery

Hideaki Nishimori, Takashi Fukutomi, Seiichiro Wariishi, Masaki Yamamoto, and Shiro Sasaguri

Purpose: We had proposed a novel therapeutic strategy against central baroreflex failure: implementation of an artificial baroreflex system to automatically regulate sympathetic vasomotor tone, i. e., a bionic baroreflex system (BBS), and tested its efficacy in a model of sudden hypotension during orthopaedic surgery. In present study we utilized a BBS during an abdominal aortic aneurysm surgery to treat hypotension occurred when declamping an aorta.

Method: Ten patients (73–84 years old, 7 males) who underwent abdominal aortic aneurysm repair were enrolled. The BBS consisted of a computer-controlled negative feedback circuit that sensed arterial pressure (AP) and automatically computed the frequency (STM) of a pulse train required to stimulate sympathetic nerves via an epidural catheter placed at the level of the lower thoracic spinal cord.

Results: Without the implementation of the BBS, a sudden declamping an aorta resulted in 15 mmHg decrease in AP within several seconds. During real-time execution of the BBS, mean AP has increased to 60 mmHg within 30 seconds. Any complications related to the BBS have not occurred.

Conclusion: In an abdominal aortic aneurysm surgery, the feasibility of a BBS approach was confirmed.

H. Nishimori, T. Fukutomi, S. Wariishi, M. Yamamoto, and S. Sasaguri
Department of Surgery 2, Kochi University, Kochi, Japan

A Case of Two Inflammatory Aortic Aneurysms Showing Spontaneous Improvement of the First Aneurysm During Development of the Second One

Yuiichi Tamori, Koichi Akutsu, Tsuyoshi Yoshimuta, Shingo Sakamoto, Toshiya Okajima, Masahiro Higashi, Hitoshi Ogino, Hiroshi Nonogi, and Satoshi Takeshita

A 66-year-old man presented with severe abdominal pain which had lasted for 2 days. Computed tomographic (CT) scanning revealed infrarenal abdominal aortic aneurysm (AAA) with a thick soft tissue around aortic walls (mantle sign). Based on the CT finding, the diagnosis was made as inflammatory AAA. Eighteen months later, due to a left hydrocele, the patient received a follow-up CT scan, which revealed spontaneous improvement of AAA with disappearance of mantle sign. It was also documented a newly developed thoracoabdominal aortic aneurysm (TAAA) associated with mantle sign. Loboratory findings revealed slightly elevated levels of erysrocyte sedimentstion rate (17 mm/hr) and fibrinogen (399 mg/dl). An 18F-labeled deoxyglucose (FDG) positron emission tomography (PET) scan showed no FDG uptake in AAA but in TAAA. Subsequent development of two inflammatory aortic aneurysms is rare. In this case, during the development of the second aneurysm, the first one spontaneously improved. The consequence of these two aneurysms suggests that inflammatory reaction associated with this disease may be a local rather than systemic pathology.

Y. Tamori, K. Akutsu, T. Yoshimuta, S. Sakamoto, T. Okajima, H. Nonogi, and S. Takeshita
Department of Cardiovascular Medicine, National Cardiovascular Center, Suita, Japan

M. Higashi
Department of Radiology, National Cardiovascular Center, Suita, Japan

H. Ogino
Department of Cardiovascular Surgery, National Cardiovascular Center, Suita, Japan

Tubercular Pseudoaneurysms of Aorta and its Branches

Shiv Kumar Choudhary, Sachin Talwar, Balram Airan,
Srikrishna Reddy, and Sanjeev Sharma

Introduction: Mycobacterial infection is a rare but definite cause of pseudoaneurysms of aorta and its branches worldwide in association with acquired immunodeficiency syndrome and drug-resistant tuberculosis (TB).

Patients and Methods: In the last decade, we treated 28 pseudoaneurysms of the aorta and its branches in 27 patients. All had evidence of treated or active TB (History of active or treated pulmonary TB, n=23, meningeal TB, n=1, military TB, n=1, treated abdominal TB, n=1, and treated cuteneous TB, n=1). 11 patients had radiological or laboratory evidence of TB. Almost all parts of aorta were involved, commonest being distal arch (n=6) and suprarenal abdominal aorta (n=6). In 3 patients, innominate artery and in one the left common carotid artery was involved. Twenty four patients underwent surgery. Histopathological examination revealed granulomatous inflammation in six patients. Four patients had positive culture for acid-fast bacilli. All patients received anti-TB chemotherapy following surgery.

Results: There were two hospital deaths: one at operation and other due to refractory meningeal TB. One patient developed recurrence at the original site after 8 months and died at re-operation.

Conclusion: Mycobacterial infection has emerged as a definite aetiology for mycotic aneurysms of the aorta and its branches.

S.K. Choudhary, S. Talwar, B. Airan, S. Reddy, and S. Sharma
Cardiothoracic and Vascular Surgery, All India Institute of Medical Sciences,
New Delhi, Republic of India

Strategy for Treating Aneurysms in the Distal Arch Aorta-open Surgery and Endovascular Repair with Single-branched Inoue Stent-graft

Hideyuki Shimizu, Naritaka Kimura, Misato Kobayashi,
Nobuko Tano, Yasuko Miyaki, Tatsuo Takahashi, Kentaro Yamabe,
Subaru Hashimoto, Yukio Kuribayashi, Kanji Inoue, and Ryohei Yozu

Summary We reviewed 155 patients who had undergone elective surgical or endovascular repair of aneurysms in the distal aortic arch. The early and late results were satisfactory regardless of therapeutic modality. Endovascular aneurysm repair for such lesions with the Inoue single-branched stent-graft seems to be a promising and valuable supplement to surgery especially for high-risk patients, although further and larger studies are needed to confirm this supposition.

Keywords aortic arch aneurysm · total arch replacement · branched stent-graft · endovascular aneurysm repair · Inoue stent-graft

Introduction

The clinical results of open surgery for aortic arch aneurysms are improving, although it is invasive and associated with high mortality and morbidity rates. On the other hand, endovascular aneurysm repair (EVAR) is less invasive. However, the indication for EVAR for aortic aneurysms in distal aortic arch is restricted, mainly because of anatomical features. The major branch vessels require special consideration. The Inoue single-branched stent-graft [1] allows reconstruction of the subclavian artery and might overcome the disadvantages of conventional stent-grafts. We retrospectively reviewed our experience with open surgery and endovascular repair using the Inoue single-branched stent-graft for distal arch aortic aneurysms.

Materials and Methods

Between 2000 and 2007, 155 patients who underwent elective surgical or endovascular treatment for aneurysms in the distal aortic arch were assigned to 3 groups based upon therapeutic modality. Our standard procedure is total arch replacement through median sternotomy under hypothermic circulatory arrest with selective antegrade cerebral perfusion. Group A comprised 122 patients who were treated with the standard procedure. The modified Bentall operation (6), valve-sparing root replacement (1), aortic valve replacement (3), mitral valve replacement (1) and coronary artery bypass grafting (29) were concomitantly performed. When the aneurysm was mainly located in the descending aorta, and when proximal cross-clamping between the left carotid and the left subclavian arteries was achievable, prosthetic graft replacement proceeded through left thoracotomy. Group B comprised 27 patients who underwent this procedure. Six patients (group C), all of whom were at high risk for conventional surgical repair because of advanced age or coexisting morbidity, and three of whom were octogenarians, underwent EVAR with the branched Inoue stent-graft. Each stent-graft was custom-made and individually designed based on information obtained by helical CT with 3D vascular reconstruction and multiplanar reconstruction. The stent-graft is delivered from the femoral artery under general anesthesia and deployed using the tug-of-wire method. The free end of the traction wire attached to the tip of the branched graft is caught by a gooseneck snare wire, which is inserted percutaneously through the left brachial artery, and the branched graft is pulled into the left subclavian artery. A balloon catheter is finally inserted into the stent-graft and inflated to stabilize the graft. Table 1 shows the preoperative characteristics of the patient.

Table 1

	Group A Median sternotomy (n=122)	Group B Left thoracotomy (n=27)	Group C EAVR (n=6)
Age	66.3 ± 10.1 (29~80)	59.9 ± 14.5 (27~78)	76.5 ± 7.6 (62~84)
M/F	81/31	16/11	6/0
EuroSCORE (Logistic)	13.2 ± 7.4%	7.5 ± 5.4%	20.6 ± 14.5%
Etiology			
Atheorosclerotic	96	8	4
Dissection	21	16	1
Pseudoaneurysm	2	1	1
Others	3 (True + Dissection)	2 (True + Dissection)	0
Diameter of aneurysm	58 ± 9 mm	57 ± 9 mm	61 ± 15 mm

Table 2

	Group A Median sternotomy (n = 122)	Group B Left thoracotomy (n = 27)	Group C EVAR (n = 6)
Operation time (minutes)	466 ± 153	315 ± 112	366 ± 75
No blood transfusion	13% (16)	56% (15)	50% (3)
Respiratory support (days)	2.6 ± 3.0	0.9 ± 0.5	0.2 ± 0.4
Mortality	3.3%	2.4%	0%
Morbidity	Cerebral infarction 2 Renal dysfunction 4	Cerebral infarction 1 Chyrothorax 1 Duodenal ulcer 1	Duodenal ulcer 1 Renal dysfunction 1

Table 3

	Group A Median sternotomy (n = 118)	Group B Left thoracotomy (n = 26)	Group C EAVR (n = 6)
Late morality	8	1	0
Aneurysm related mortality	3 (rupture 2, sudden death 1)	0	0
Graft failure	0	0	0
Endoleak	N/A	N/A	0
Aneurysm expansion	N/A	N/A	0

Results

Table 2 shows the early results of the procedures. Hospital mortality rates for groups A, B, and C were 3.3%, 2.4% and 0%, respectively. Table 3 shows the late clinical results, which were satisfactory with all procedures. Notably, neither early/late mortality nor graft failure due to causes such as endoleak or aneurysm expansion have yet occurred in any patient in group C.

Discussion

Aortic aneurysms in the distal aortic arch can be treated using several approaches. Our routine strategy of total arch replacement through median sternotomy achieves excellent results even when concomitant procedures are necessary. However, this type of surgery can be too invasive for compromised patients. Although EVAR should reduce the mortality and morbidity rates for such patients, anatomical features such as curvature of the proximal neck and the presence of branch vessels can cause difficulties that severely restrict its indications for distal arch aortic aneurysms. The innovative Inoue single-branched stent-graft is a unique, unified trunk and branch structure that does not leak at the conjunction of the module and thus can be used to treat distal arch aortic aneurysms without sacrificing a branch vessel.

Its bellows structure without a longitudinal strut allows high flexibility and high compliance for complex anatomy. Rings outside the trunk graft for hemostasis achieve high protection against leakage. Although our experience is presently limited, this innovative device might represent a significant breakthrough for treating distal arch aortic aneurysms.

Conclusions

Open surgery for the distal aortic arch achieves satisfactory early and late results. Some of these lesions can be repaired using the Inoue single-branched stent-graft with excellent short- and mid-term clinical outcomes. This innovative device seems to offer a promising and valuable supplement to surgical therapy for the distal arch aorta especially in high-risk patients, although further and larger studies are needed to confirm its effectiveness.

Reference

1. Inoue K, Hosokawa H, Iwase T, et al (1999) Aortic arch reconstruction by transluminally placed endovascular branched stent graft. Circulation 100: II-316–21

Redo Left Thoracotomy for Surgical Repair on the Descending Thoracic and Thoracoabdominal Aorta

Kenji Minatoya, Hitoshi Ogino, Hitoshi Matsuda, Hiroaki Sasaki, Hiroshi Tanaka, and Soichiro Kitamura

Objectives: Redo left thoracotomy for surgical repair on the descending thoracic and thoracoabdominal aorta is often surgical challenge. We retrospectively analyzed the outcome of the redo left thoracotomy for descending thoracic and thoracoabdominal aortic repair.

Methods: Since 2000, 25 patients underwent redo left thoracotomy for graft replacement of descending thoracic and thoracoabdominal aorta (mean age 61±13, 17 male). Thoracoabdominal aortic replacement was performed in 18 patients, and descending aortic replacement was performed in 7. There was one emergency case (4.0%). Six patients were Marfan syndrome. All operations were performed under partial cardiopulmonary bypass with segmental clamping. Preoperative MR angiography has been performed to detect Adamkiewicz artery for elective cases. Motor evoked potential has been measured to detect spinal ischemia.

Results: There was no mortality. No patient showed paraplegia and one (4.0%) showed paraparesis. The stroke rate was 0.4% (1 of 25). The rate of respiratory failure was 0.8% (2 of 25) including the patient who had stroke.

Conclusions: The redo left thoracotomy for graft replacement of descending thoracic and thoracoabdominal aorta was supposed to have more morbidity, but practically performed with an acceptable risk. The staged strategy for extensive aortic disease could be one of the surgical options.

K. Minatoya, H. Ogino, H. Matsuda, H. Sasaki, H. Tanaka, and S. Kitamura
Department of Cardiovascular Surgery, National Cardiovascular Center, Suita, Japan